FITNESS FIRST

YOUR MINDSET FOR OVERALL HEALTH, HAPPINESS, AND LIFE TRANSFORMATION

JOSHUA J GRENELL

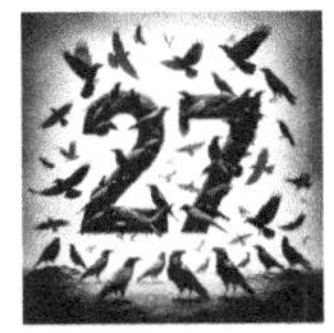

ISBN: 979-8-89504-369-1

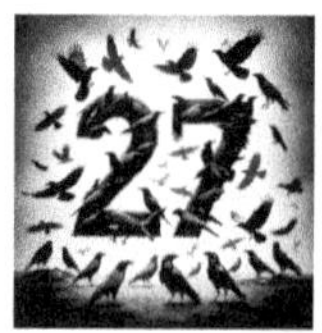

27 Crows Publishing

To my partner Jen, whose unwavering support and belief in me have been the bedrock of my journey, this book is dedicated with all my love and gratitude. To my family, who have fueled my drive and ambition, I owe a debt of gratitude that words cannot express. To Nicholas Scudamore and Julianne O'Brien, who have allowed me the time to write this book through their dedication and hard work. I am profoundly thankful to the incredible members of Progression Fitness whose commitment, resilience and camaraderie have inspired this book and shaped the essence of my being. Lastly, to all those who have walked with me, guided me, and supported me through various stages of my life. This book is a tribute to all of you who have made Fitness First a title and a lived reality. Thank you for being my strength, inspiration, and reason to strive for greatness. Lastly, I thank Chris Cooper, who showed me the path to many things—writing this book is among them.

CONTENTS

Over the past five years, a journey of profound personal research and evolution unfolded. This book, *Fitness First*, is the culmination of countless hours of reflection, research, and real-life experiences, all of which converged toward a singular realization. The path to its creation was anything but linear; the narrative took numerous turns, each a stepping stone contributing to its depth and purpose. It wasn't until the COVID-19 pandemic gripped the world that my focus solidified, and my ideas aligned into a coherent message.

The pandemic was a harsh mirror to society. It revealed vulnerabilities in our health systems and personal health philosophies. The closure of gyms and fitness centers worldwide created widespread frustration—an integral part of many people's daily routine was shut off.

A number of people from my gyms messaged me about their need for the gym to reopen due to their rapidly deteriorating mental health. This proved just how significant a role gyms play in many people's lives. I believe humans need movement, social connection, cooperation, belonging, and fitness—and you can find all of these things in the gym.

Unfortunately, the health benefits of fitness don't make for good marketing ads, so they are often relegated to a secondary status, overshadowed by the pursuit of "mirror fitness." Because of this, gyms are often seen as factories for sculpting abs, improving physique, and getting your cardio in. Fitness is not seen as part of health improvement and maintenance but as something you do for vanity reasons.

I see this in my daily life, where success in the gym is judged on how you look, as opposed to overall life satisfaction and health improvements. Simply put, six-pack abs do not equal health.

This realization drove me to embark on a personal journey of advocating for the mindset shift I present in this book. It's a journey I hope will inspire you to reconsider your own perceptions of fitness, health, and gyms.

MY MESSAGE IS SIMPLE: You control your health and fitness. Put your fitness first, and watch everything in your life change.

This isn't a novel concept, yet it seems increasingly forgotten in a world obsessed with superficial metrics of beauty and success. Fitness shouldn't be merely an item on our daily checklist, nor should it be pursued solely for the approval or admiration of others. Instead, it should be revered as the foundation of our lives, a nonnegotiable priority that underpins every other aspiration and achievement.

Therefore, *Fitness First* is more than just a guide to physical well-being; it's a manifesto for reclaiming control over one's health and recognizing fitness as the cornerstone of a fulfilling life. It challenges conventional narratives, urging readers to redefine their relationships with their bodies and by extension, with the very concept of health care. This book is an invitation to embark on a journey not to the perfect body but to a healthier, more empowered self.

As you turn these pages, I invite you to reflect on your own perceptions of health and fitness. My hope is that this book will be a catalyst for change, not just in how you exercise but also in how you prioritize your well-being.

Welcome to *Fitness First*, where the journey to a healthier, happier, and more helpful you begins.

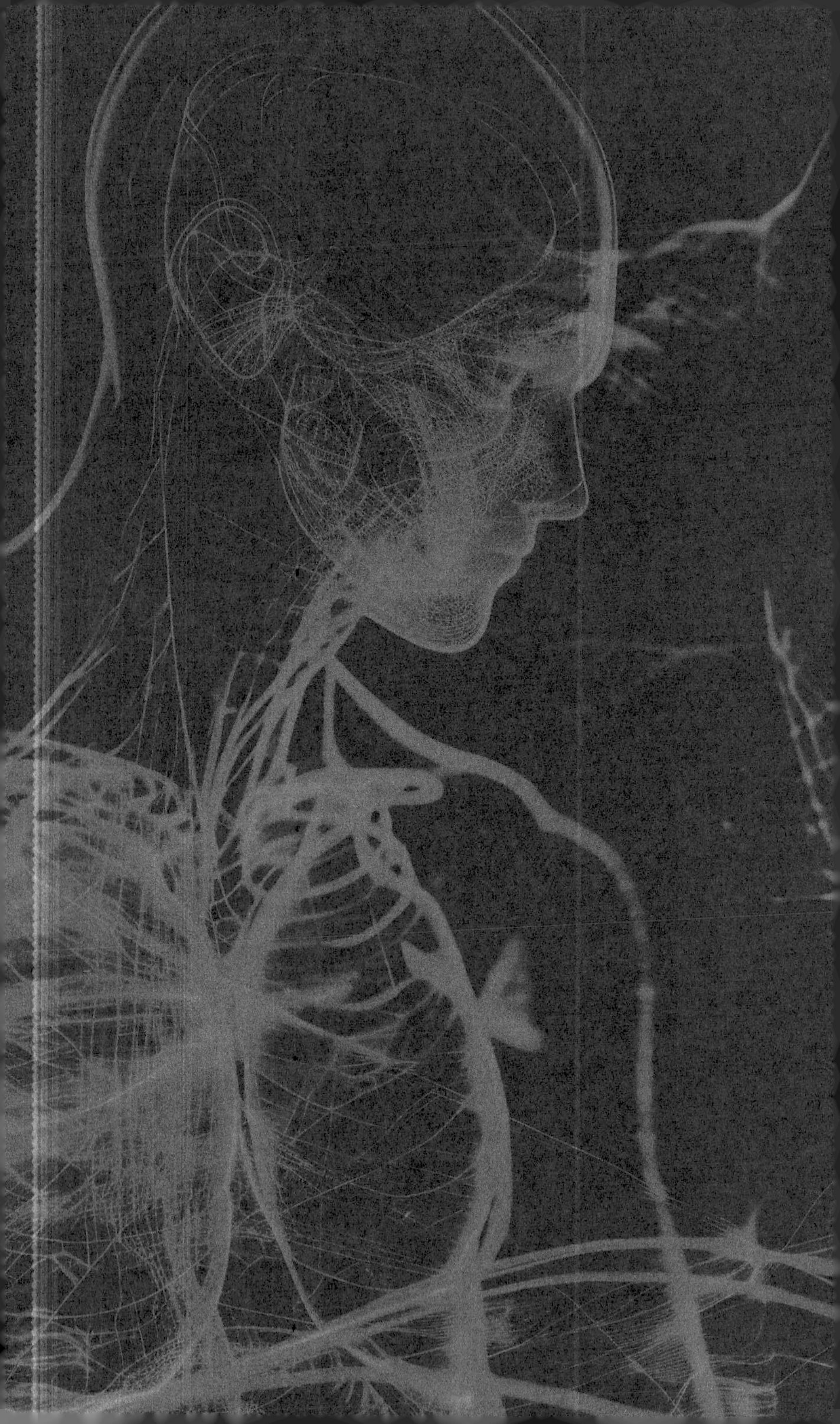

PART I

CHANGING YOUR MINDSET

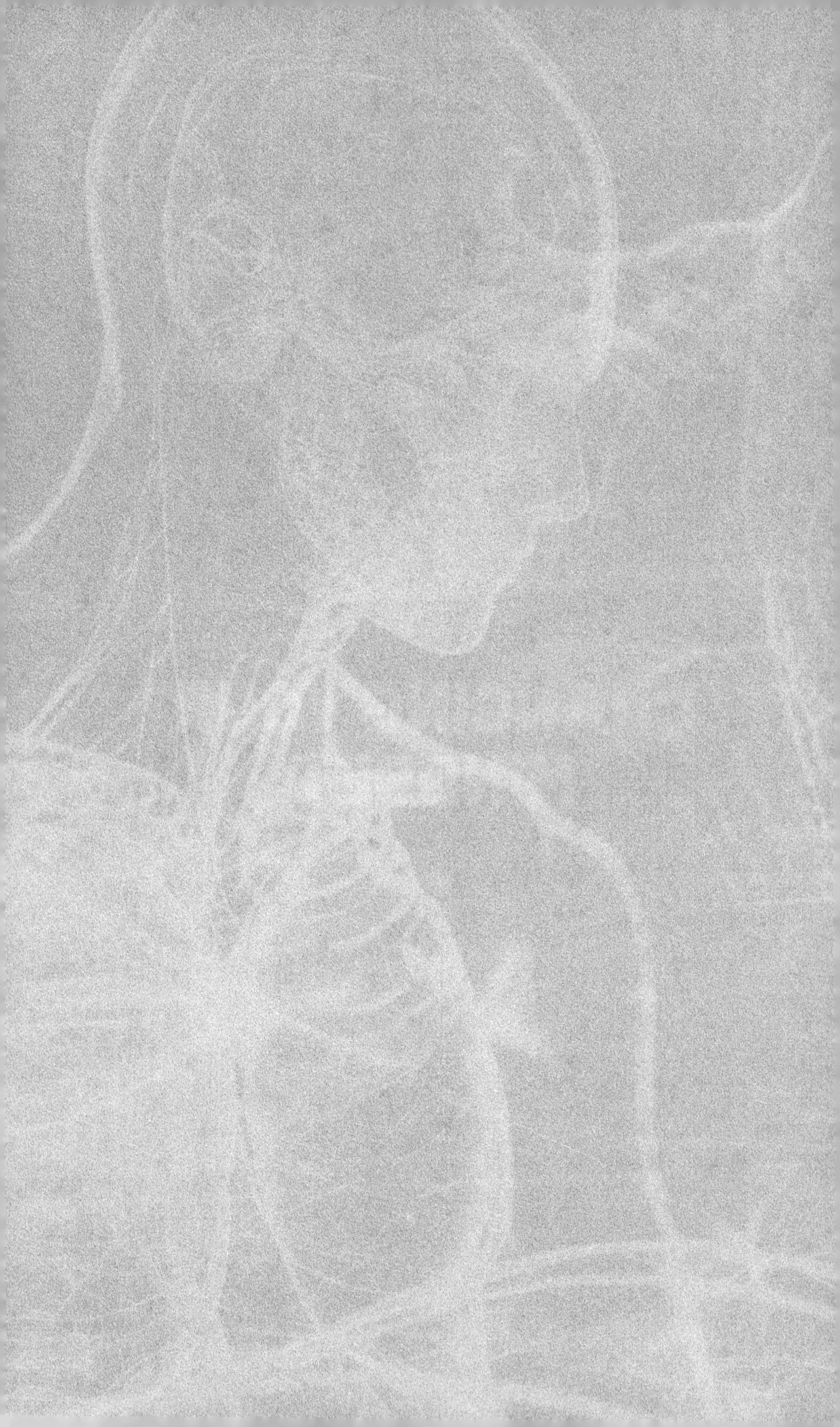

CHAPTER 1

FITNESS IS HEALTH

Changing Your Mindset from Vanity to Health

Fitness is the overall well-being of all the body's systems. It's the state where an individual feels healthy and strong, both physically and mentally. Fitness isn't just about having a toned or muscular body or performing well in physical tasks. Getting "jacked" isn't fitness, and getting "shredded" isn't healthy—even if it's sexy as hell and will garner you attention.

Recently, a friend of mine lost thirty pounds and posted about it on Facebook. Her weight loss post got more likes and engagement than when she announced the birth of her youngest child. Abs and sexy shit sells, but it is also the primary problem with how we view exercise—and possibly one of the United States' main health problems. Gyms are seen as places to get sexy, not healthy.

The misselling of fitness carries dire consequences: It's easy to stop exercising if you think it's just about looks. It isn't as easy to stop when you realize that, in reality, exercise is the most important thing you can do. Fitness is something you need to be human, participate in society, do your job, and help your family and community.

Fitness is about having healthy bodily systems that work efficiently, including cardiovascular, respiratory, muscular and nervous systems. It includes having a healthy emotional and mental state that empowers you to easily tackle life's normal challenges, leading to a healthy and fulfilling life.

According to health experts, fitness is not the same as health. Medications can make vital signs and blood work look good, even when someone's not actually fit—but any activity outside of their normal routine would expose this. How can you be considered healthy if you can't run to the aid of someone in need?

Health transcends the mere absence of illness or disease; it is a holistic state of well-being, intertwining good nutritional habits, adequate rest, and regular physical activity. Achieving perfect health may seem unattainable, but embracing a "Fitness First" mentality can significantly enhance your life, ensuring you're ready to help and be useful in everyday situations.

Consider your current lifestyle and dietary habits. Are they conducive to health and vitality? Reflect on your aspirations and life goals, and realize that achieving these is possible only with a consistent fitness routine. The reality is unavoidable: Over time, neglecting physical activity and proper nutrition may contribute to diminished quality of life and premature mortality—early death.

You can't be there for your family or friends if you are dead.

This book is your companion on your journey toward better health and fitness, helping you realize the importance of maintaining an active, nutritionally balanced lifestyle. It's not about temporary fixes or fleeting challenges—rather, instilling lifelong habits that foster functional, vibrant living. The objective is to transform your perspective on health and fitness, particularly its role in personal fulfillment and its ability to enable us to support our loved ones and make impactful contributions. By the conclusion, you'll see health and fitness as much more than mere items on a daily to-do list.

Fitness First

Your health and fitness are the most crucial aspects of your life and are worthy of your time investment. Your accomplishments, whether in your profession, interests, or connections, are reliant on your health and fitness. Your family's future success and welfare also depend on your health and fitness. Research shows that fit and healthy parents have fitter and healthier kids than those who do not exercise. What legacy are you leaving your family? Do you lead by example? Are you showing your family how to be healthy and impactful?

My Real Reason

I am writing this book for myself, my friends, and anyone who has struggled to balance health and fitness in their life. As a registered nurse and gym owner, I have met many people who need help with their fitness and health goals. I've seen firsthand the transformative impact of fitness on a person's life. I've also witnessed many people struggle and slip away from their goals, unaware of the impact their daily decisions make on their lives. This has driven me to help change people's mindsets toward exercise.

Fitness First Is a Mindset

Adopting a fitness-oriented mindset is an acquired skill, not an inherent instinct. Throughout my journey, I've experienced several key moments that profoundly shaped my outlook on health and well-being, illuminating the critical role that fitness plays across all facets of life: personal, professional, and social. But mastering the application of this philosophy and sharing it with others was a journey in itself.

My family's medical history greatly influenced my commitment to a health-centric lifestyle. My grandfather's life was cut short by a heart attack at thirty-nine, a fate that nearly befell my father at 46. His stark warning about the inevitability of another potentially fatal heart attack is a memory that has never left me, and that period marked a pivotal chapter in my life. Witnessing the vulnerability of my loved ones propelled me into action, and health, fitness, and the pursuit of longevity became my core passions. This book is designed to guide you toward becoming the healthiest version of yourself, as you recognize the transformative power of prioritizing fitness amidst life's challenges.

Are You Fit Enough?

Many individuals need help grasping the critical role of fitness in their daily lives. While aware of the need to exercise, it rarely becomes a priority and is frequently not included in their weekly agendas. Instead, it is an "if I have time" thing.

Many members of my gyms achieve remarkable fitness gains quickly, yet some take these improvements for granted, oblivious to their enhanced state of health. When we host events for friends and family, these often serve as eye-openers for newcomers who struggle with even the basic warm-up routines. Our regular members are shocked that something they now see as easy is so hard for their friends who seem "in shape." This highlights the substantial fitness disparities between them, as well as the considerable impact of regular exercise–even on those who outwardly appeared healthy already. These differences become apparent when people are put in positions to use their fitness. Remember, blood draws and the scale may suggest you are fit, even if the reality differs.

Gym members' decisions to discontinue their fitness regimens concern me deeply, not just as a gym owner but as a health advocate. The justifications I hear—from financial commitments to personal milestones—reflect a misunderstanding of the fundamental value of health and fitness. Sadly, some individuals neglect their well-being for material or economic reasons, a choice that has dire consequences on their health and longevity. In the big picture, stopping your gym membership to purchase a new car or bigger house is a very poor decision.

Exercise is far more than an item on a to-do list. It's a cornerstone of healthy living and longevity. You are made for movement and activity. Neglecting this natural inclination can lead to detrimental health outcomes in many areas. Not moving is bad for you—and it is bad for you quickly.

A two-week break from regular movement significantly reduces lean muscle mass, cardiovascular endurance, and insulin sensitivity. After just two weeks, you start to get unhealthy. Further, a study from Biomed Central[1] found that after two months of not training, elite athletes showed unfavorable changes in body composition, impaired metabolic function, and development of cardio-vascular risk factors.

How fast your health and fitness deteriorates depends on how fit you are and how long you have been exercising. The longer you have exercised con-sistently, the slower its health benefits disappear.

Exercise has a building block effect on your body. The more consistently you work out, the more resilient you become to life's curveballs. This fact is displayed in the diagram below, adapted from one I first saw at a CrossFit Level 1 seminar[2] in 2008. This lone diagram inspired me to open my first gym.

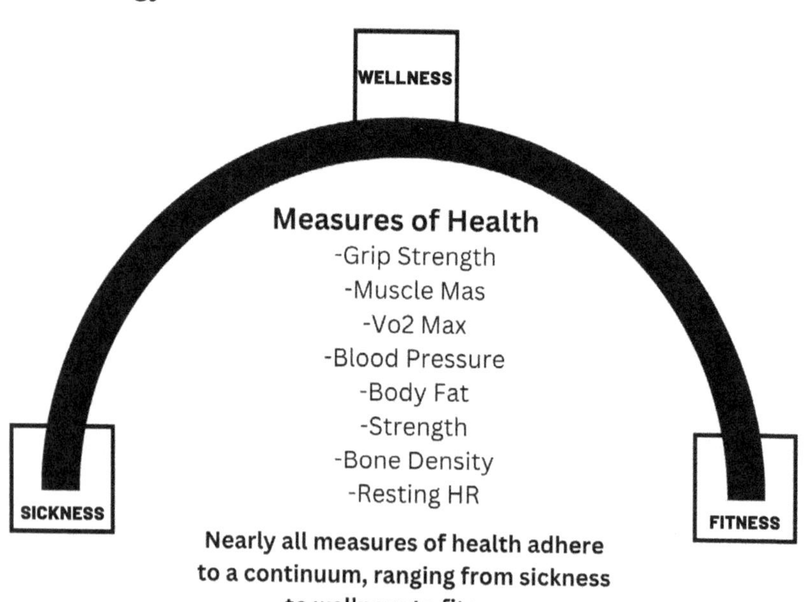

Nearly all measures of health adhere to a continuum, ranging from sickness to wellness to fitness.

Consistency Is King

A consistent exercise routine acts as a protective barrier for your health. Within just two weeks of halting gym visits, many individuals experience a weight gain of five to ten pounds, as well as a noticeable decrease in their work capacity. This process accelerates with age and has significant negative implications.

When members leave the gym, only a tiny fraction persist toward their fitness goals. Even if they continue to exercise, work out independently, or explore new physical activities, most fail to remain consistent.

Getting Restarted Sucks

Reintegrating into your gym routine presents considerable challenges. Fitness is slowly gained but quickly lost, often making the journey back to prior fitness levels painful and protracted. The longer you went to the gym previously, the longer it will take you to get back to where you were. This slow return to your previous fitness often results in discouragement, leading many to abandon their efforts with the mistaken belief that they can no longer achieve their fitness goals.

However, the notion that it's too late to enhance one's fitness is fundamentally flawed. Regular, appropriate exercise can significantly impact individuals of any age. In today's world, it's not uncommon to find individuals over seventy engaging in various activities at gyms, challenging the misconception that age is a barrier to maintaining an active lifestyle. These seniors defy traditional expectations of aging and exemplify the potential to remain active in hiking, sports, family activities, and personal projects. They often become role models in their communities, demonstrating that strength and vitality can extend well into the later years and establishing a new normal for aging with grace and vigor.

Find Your Real Reason

Is it possible to continue engaging in activities you enjoy, regardless of age? This question takes on different meanings at various stages of life and plays a pivotal role in your overall happiness and sense of fulfillment. Aging doesn't mandate a cessation of cherished activities or that you resign yourself to dependency on others.

Maintaining independence means you don't have to relinquish your role in supporting family, friends, and neighbors. Your travel plans don't need to be constrained by physical limitations, nor must your home maintenance depend on hiring outside help—unless gardening and lawn care aren't your cup of tea. Imagine still being able to shoot hoops with your children, embark on cycling adventures, care for your grandchildren, or rearrange furniture well into your eighties. This is the essence of Fitness First.

Caring for yourself enables you to be there for your loved ones more effectively. After all, you can only truly offer assistance when you're in good health. Embracing a Fitness First mindset means recognizing that peak mental and physical condition is crucial for excelling in various areas of life that demand energy and attention. Eventually, everyone faces physical limitations, but your goal should be to delay these restrictions as long as possible, enhancing your quality of life and extending your active years—not just for you but also for those you care about.

During a recent visit to Yellowstone National Park, something odd struck me. Despite the crowds that thronged the main roads, venturing just a short distance on foot revealed a starkly empty landscape. Individuals in their thirties to fifties seemed unable or unwilling to walk even 200 feet to an observation deck. Some parents opted to stay in their cars, sending only their children to explore. This experience shed light on the alarming state of physical fitness among many visitors.

Choosing to prioritize health and fitness can revolutionize your quality of life. Beyond just enhancing vacation experiences, it allows you to reclaim the ability to engage in everyday activities—an ability many lose too soon due to preventable conditions. A staggering number of parents find themselves sidelined from actively participating in their children's lives, not due to incurable diseases but due to lifestyle choices that are within their power to change.

Moreover, some manage well on the surface but falter when faced with physical challenges. A seemingly benign hike or a casual game of ultimate frisbee can abruptly expose a person's fitness shortcomings. I encountered such wake-up calls in my late twenties, struggling on a mountain bike ride and feeling overwhelmed during a sports game. I was that guy who looked healthy but could not perform. But these experiences aren't signals to resign or give up; they're signals to embrace change and get going.

Engaging actively with your children or enjoying daily activities may not seem like high-stakes performances, and being able to continue doing what you love for as long as possible may not be the most glamorous motivator—but it is a valid reason to prioritize your fitness. We will explore your reason further in chapter four.

CHAPTER 2

INSPIRATIONAL FITNESS STORIES

According to research from the Centers for Disease Control and Prevention,[3] physical activity is the most important thing humans can do for their well-being and fitness. Exercising regularly produces various health benefits, such as reducing blood pressure levels, improving cholesterol levels, minimizing the risk of type 2 diabetes and metabolic syndrome, reducing the risk of various cancers, improving your mental health, and increasing your chances of living longer. And it also makes you feel good.

You Can Only Do What You Love If You Are Fit

Most of us have a lot of things we want to do, and being fit enough to do them is essential. For instance, you can't volunteer to build houses to help the less fortunate if you're not fit enough to do manual labor. You can't help your mom with her household tasks as she ages if you're unable to walk a flight of stairs without shortness of breath.

Some of the more alarming questions we must ask ourselves involve whether we're able to protect our family and ourselves by performing well in an emergency: If your child is wandering into heavy traffic and you are twenty yards away, can you reach them in time? And if you get to them, will you be okay, or will you need help due to the exertion you just exhibited? How long could you survive if you were caught in a flood and had to hang on for your life? Could you get your kids out of your house during a fire? Could you stop someone from taking your child from you?

These may seem like extreme examples, but they are worth considering. It's important to be honest with yourself when answering these questions.

Things We Love to Do

We all have things we love to do, and many of them are active in some way. You may enjoy yardwork or gardening, or you may love to golf. You may enjoy taking care of your grandchildren or walking your dog. Maybe you love to work, and your work requires you to be physically able to perform manual tasks. Putting Fitness First can add years to these activities.

To illustrate this, I'll share a story about a remarkable woman who truly left an impression on me. While browsing Facebook, I came across an ad for Japanese maples. The deal seemed too good to pass up—I'd been eyeing these maples for a while. When I arrived at the woman's house to collect them, I was taken aback by the beauty of her yard. It was a living masterpiece, dotted with quaint gardens and flower beds, straight out of a glossy home and garden magazine. She was in her early sixties and exuded health and vitality. She had prepped the three large trees for me, all potted and ready for their new home.

What struck me the most was her story. She shared that she had been wrestling with cancer for the last three years, a battle that had sapped her strength, making it challenging to tend to her beloved trees and garden. Yet, here she was, determined to care for her green sanctuary as much as her body would permit. Reluctantly, she decided to part with some of her plants, ensuring they went to someone who could provide the care she no longer could.

Her resilience was inspiring. Her dedication to her gardens never wavered despite facing every reason to step back. Gardening wasn't just a hobby for her; it was a lifeline, a physical activity that kept her moving and as healthy as possible. This encounter was a powerful reminder of how our passions deeply intertwine with our well-being. It also reminded me of how vital our physical abilities are to our passions.

Another notable example is that of Marcy and John, a couple whose story is closely connected to the heart of our gym's community. They began their fitness journey just as John was close to retiring from IBM. John's goal was to canoe from their home all the way down the Mississippi. I am not sure what Marcy's goal was when they first started together, but she had a rough start. She was one of those people who looked healthy on the exterior but was quickly exposed when the activities started. But Marcy is now probably one of the fittest people in her age group in our city due to her consistency.

Over a decade has passed since they first walked through our gym's doors. In that time, Marcy has emerged as a pillar of strength, achieving feats she once thought impossible. Her transformation enabled her to support John in more ways than one, even lending a hand in his workshop with tasks that demanded physical prowess. Together, they reached milestones many only dream of: mastering pull-ups and setting an inspiring example for their peers.

John's journey, in particular, is a testament to the power of perseverance. His health flourished, with significant improvements that saw his vital signs managed and vastly improved. His vitality enabled him to outperform men half his age, a sight I witnessed firsthand.

It is with a heavy heart that we now remember John. Recently, he was taken from us in a tragic event, leaving a void in our community and Marcy's life. His legacy, however, endures in the strength and determination he displayed, in the goals he achieved, and in the love and camaraderie he fostered within our gym family. As we continue to support Marcy, we honor John's memory, cherishing his inspiration and the journey he shared with us all. Here is John's Hero workout:

- ► "JC" Hero Workout
- ► 7 rounds for time:
- ► 8 kettlebell swings
- ► 22 push-ups
- ► 5 strict pull-ups
- ► 1,000-meter row (800-meter run)

A final inspiring fitness journey I'd like to spotlight is Cally's. Cally has been with our gym for more than eight years, after retiring from a successful career in the insurance industry. She stands out not just as a great member but as an incredible grandmother, boasting fitness levels that allow her to run around with her grandchildren without missing a beat.

Her journey hasn't been without its challenges: Cally has had major health concerns. Yet, her commitment to regular workouts has turned the tide, significantly helping her through her health issues. Her doctor's orders? Keep up the great work; the exercise regimen she's been following has made a difference. Cally's story is a testament to the impact of fitness on quality of life.

Things We Do for Our Loved Ones

Other older adults start exercise programs because they notice decreased function or abilities. This serves as a wake-up call, often not one of concern for yourself but for your loved ones.

One of the best stories I have heard is the story of a grandmother who was watching her grandchild when the child started running into the street. The grandmother could not stop the child, and this inability flipped the switch: She decided to make herself a better grandparent by exercising. The need to function enough to watch and protect your grandchildren is powerful.

For her, starting to exercise wasn't about extending her life—that's an additional benefit. Her main reason was to expand her ability to function, enjoy life, and be responsible for her family.

Another significant story is from my childhood when our family friends were victims of a home invasion. A man and woman broke into their home and attempted to gain control of the homeowners. They tied up the husband and started to tie up his wife. Fortunately, the wife, whom we will call Sue, was fit enough to attack and win a fight with the two using only a frying pan. Later, my family loaned them a handgun, so they could feel safer at home, and I remember asking my dad why they needed a gun when they had Sue!

The stories of the importance of fitness are endless. For most people, it is simply about getting the most out of their life. Countless gym members have told me stories about enjoying life more, such as "You know, Josh, when we go on vacation, we like to do stuff. Most people our age can't do much, but thanks to the gym, we do everything. We hang out with the twenty-year-olds all day!" A lot of people think they could never do those kinds of activities, but the reality is that anyone can improve their fitness, no matter their age.

Are You Fit Enough to Do Your Job?

Have you ever had one of those moments where you ask yourself, "Am I fit enough to be doing what I'm doing?" And I'm not just talking about opening tight jars, running to catch the bus, or climbing stairs that suddenly feel like Mount Everest. I'm also referring to things like mental sharpness, problem-solving skills, and having the stamina to tackle the daily grind and keep going when your bed is calling.

Have you ever noticed that you're a genius after a morning run? That's not just you being awesome; it's science. Exercising in the morning supercharges your brainpower for hours. Our brains are pretty greedy when it comes to energy, so the extra blood flow from getting your heart rate up acts like an octane boost straight to your brain cells.

Being fit isn't just about being able to flex in the mirror or outrun your neighbor's dog. It's about being mentally and physically ready for whatever life throws. I've worked many jobs where I wasn't sure the guy next to me was up to the task if I needed him. Don't be that guy.

Even worse than not being fit for your job is not being around to do your job. You can't do your job if you're six feet under. Incredible people are doing great things, but sometimes, they're stopped in their tracks way too soon because their health wasn't on their priority list. I knew a fantastic teacher who was making a huge impact and then was suddenly gone at fifty-two. The loss was felt far beyond just family and friends; the community lost a spark that can't be replaced, and many kids and families will miss out on knowing her.

Back when I worked at the Mayo Clinic, my unit was a fair distance from the main hospital, so when the security team was called in for emergencies, it was a bit of a jog to get to us. Whenever we needed help, which was often, security would show up in stages. The fit ones were the first to arrive; they were ready to go and made a real difference. Once the others got there, sometimes they couldn't catch their breath enough to help.

Think about it: No matter what your job is—cop, firefighter, soldier—you want someone by your side who's got their act together, physically and mentally. Nobody hopes for a teammate who will lag behind when the going gets tough.

The moral of this chapter is to take care of yourself. Fitness isn't a luxury; it's a necessity for performing at our best, handling the pressures of life, and being there for those who count on us. From personal anecdotes to professional observations, it's clear that fitness can mean the difference between success or failure and even life or death.

As we head into the next chapter, remember: Exercise isn't just about looks or setting a personal record; it's about living your life to the fullest, tackling your job like a boss, and being there for the people counting on you. And hey, if you look good in your jeans, consider it a bonus.

Now, let's take a look into that brain of yours.

THE MIND-BODY CONNECTION

Understanding the Biological Link between Exercise and the Mind

Physical activity and mental health are connected by a complex biochemical dance. When we exercise, our body releases a cocktail of neurotransmitters and hormones, such as endorphins, dopamine, norepinephrine, and serotonin. These chemicals are pivotal in regulating mood, anxiety, and stress levels. Endorphins, often referred to as the body's natural painkillers, also induce feelings of euphoria and well-being, a state sometimes known as the "runner's high." This high is available to all of us—even those of us who don't run.

The impact of physical activity on mental health is not limited to the immediate release of these feel-good chemicals. Regular exercise has been shown to contribute to long-term improvements in brain health, including enhancements in neuroplasticity and the brain's ability to form new neural connections. This is critical for cognitive function, learning, and memory. Moreover, physical activity can act as a powerful counterbalance to the effects of stress, reducing the physical and mental wear and tear associated with chronic stress exposure.

Exercise as a Tool for Mental Health Disorders

The therapeutic benefits of exercise extend into the realm of clinical mental health conditions, such as anxiety, depression, ADHD, and PTSD. For individuals grappling with anxiety and stress, even short bursts of physical activity can serve as an effective antidote, helping to lower immediate symptoms of anxiety and reduce stress over time. The benefits for depression are equally compelling, with research suggesting that regular physical activity can be as effective as medication or psychotherapy for some individuals.

Attention-deficit/hyperactivity disorder (ADHD) and post-traumatic stress disorder (PTSD) may also see significant benefits from regular physical engagement. For ADHD, exercise improves concentration, motivation, and mood, akin to the effects of traditional ADHD medications. This is due to increased dopamine and norepinephrine levels, crucial for attention and executive functioning. PTSD, on the other hand, can be alleviated through exercise by helping individuals become more attuned to their bodily sensations, aiding the process of re-establishing a sense of control over their physical state—a technique known as "grounding."

Age-Specific Benefits and Guidelines

I have a bonus chapter at the end of this book specifically addressing age and exercise goals. The positive impacts of physical activity span all ages, with specific benefits and recommendations tailored to each life stage.

For children and adolescents, regular physical engagement is not only crucial for physical development but also for mental and emotional health. It fosters self-esteem, reduces the risk of depression, and can improve academic performance. The World Health Organization[4] recommends that children and adolescents spend at least sixty minutes per day engaging in moderate-to-vigorous intensity physical activity, mainly aerobic.

Adults, including the elderly, can also reap significant mental health benefits from regular physical activity. WHO recommends they engage in a weekly minimum of 150 to 300 minutes of moderate-intensity or seventy-five to 150 minutes of vigorous-intensity aerobic exercise, or a combination of both. For older adults, physical activity is linked to improved mood and cognitive function, enhanced functional capacity, and reduced risk of falls.

A Holistic Approach to Mental Health

Embracing physical activity as a cornerstone of mental health requires a shift in how we perceive the role of exercise in our lives—this is the main premise of this book. Exercise is not merely a strategy for managing weight or physical health conditions but a fundamental component of mental and emotional well-being. By fostering a culture that values and promotes physical activity, we can unlock its full potential as a powerful, accessible means of enhancing mental health, improving quality of life, and building resilience against the challenges of modern life.

The conversation around mental health and physical activity also acknowledges the inherent interconnectivity of the human mind and body. Recognizing that one cannot thrive without the other shifts the paradigm from treating mental and physical health in isolation to a more integrated, holistic approach.

Physical activity, in its myriad forms, offers a unique avenue to combat and prevent a range of mental health conditions. The evidence is clear: From reducing symptoms of anxiety and depression to enhancing cognitive function and emotional well-being across all age groups, the benefits are vast and significant. Exercise should be the first priority in everyone's life.

But the journey doesn't stop with individual action. Societal attitudes and structures are crucial in facilitating or hindering access to physical activity. Urban planning that prioritizes pedestrian-friendly spaces, public policies that support community sports programs, and workplaces that encourage active breaks are examples of systemic changes that can foster a culture of movement.

Moreover, healthcare providers and mental health professionals are increasingly recognizing the value of incorporating physical activity into treatment plans for mental health conditions. This doesn't mean exercise is a substitute for professional mental health care when needed. Rather, it is a complementary approach that can significantly enhance the effectiveness of traditional treatments. I can't tell you how many times taking a walk around the unit helped my psychiatric patients deal with what they were experiencing. There were days when I logged 30,000 or more steps in a twelve-hour shift. Walking may not fix depression, but it certainly helps the brain get back on track.

Education is another critical component. Raising awareness about the mental health benefits of physical activity can motivate individuals to incorporate more movement into their daily lives. Schools, in particular, have a unique opportunity to instill the importance of physical activity from an early age, equipping children with knowledge and habits that can support their mental health throughout their lives. But instead, it seems we are moving the opposite direction, getting rid of physical education and exercise in schools. While our kids get more and more unhealthy, we cut programs that are known to help.

Embracing physical activity is about improving physical health and nurturing our mental and emotional well-being. Physical activities profoundly impact mental health–this is grounded in scientific research and supplemented by practical advice for integrating movement into daily life.

The path to a healthier mind is through the body; every movement brings us closer to better health and fitness. The journey toward improved mental health through physical activity is one of empowerment, resilience, and collective action.

Next, let's look at motivation and how improving it can make a real difference to ourselves and those around us.

CHAPTER 4

FINDING YOUR PERSONAL MOTIVATION

Everyone Needs a Goal

"Goals" are an individual's desired results and outcomes, including personal goals, professional goals, fitness goals, career goals, and many more. The key to achieving these goals is the reason behind them. Staying motivated is hard when circumstances or the environment around you become unsupportive or indifferent, but if you have a resilient mindset about your goals and the reason behind the goal is powerful enough, you are unstoppable.

Working toward your goals can be challenging in today's world, which is full of chaos, distractions, and competition. Setting a general or non-specific goal won't be enough in this environment. To get through this challenging environment, you must have a powerful "why." General and non-specific goals are why most people's New Year's Resolutions are bound for failure. You must set specific goals and identify why you want to achieve them.

Fitness Goals

Embarking toward the journey of a fitness-first lifestyle requires an individual to set clear fitness goals and know the real reason behind each goal. Those reasons will become the source of their motivation and act as a rescue device or way of continuing through any situation until they have accomplished that goal.

The goals society has flashed at us since the beginning of advertising are designed to make you buy something—and they do work to that end. You buy what they want you to, but the results don't come. And if they do come, they don't stay. These societal goals have never been able to change any individual's long-term behavior.

For instance, wanting six-pack abs may get you into the gym, but it will only keep you there for a short time. Keeping you active requires a more profound reason and a determined mindset.

Superficial, top-level goals don't work because they only touch the surface level of an individual's goals; they must be deeper to provide the push required to get through times when motivation is low.

Here are some examples of deeper reasons:

- ▶ I want to become fit because I need to get healthier and be more attractive to find my mate.

- ▶ I am a shadow of my true self, so I want to see my capabilities and strengths.

- ▶ I want to get fit because I cannot keep up with my children.

- ▶ I am afraid I might die.

Getting to your real reason gives you power. It offers you the extra push to get you out of bed and to help you turn your life around. Even the reasons above may need to be deeper. Often, people join gyms with superficial goals in their minds, without any deeper reasons or motivation to achieve them. They have goals, but they need to be more specific and deeper.

Here are some common goals and ways to improve them:

"I am going to get to the gym three times a week from now on."

- ► Most people need help determining the real reason behind this decision. How long will they do it? Why have they chosen a limit of three times per week? What will they do once they are at the gym? How will they measure if it is working? What does success look like? Without these questions answered, most people will find themselves in no better situation in six months than when they started.

"I want to get healthy!"

- ► The main questions here are: Why do you want to get healthy? How will you know when you are healthy? And who will benefit from this change in your life? You must find your true motivation for making such changes, even if it means digging beneath the surface goal to uncover your reason. Again, what does "healthy" mean? How will you know if you've reached it? And why does that matter?

"I want to lose weight!"

► This goal is most prevalent among those who join gyms. Whenever these people are asked why they want to lose weight, they usually struggle to answer. I hear things like "So I can fit in my clothes," "I have put on a few pounds recently due to work," and "Doesn't everyone want to lose weight?" People give a lot of answers to the "Why do you want to lose weight?" question, but rarely is the answer enough to get them to their goals.

Weight loss is a superficial goal. Wanting to lose weight will not get you out of bed when the alarm goes off in the morning, and it will not make you turn right toward the gym instead of heading home after work. It isn't enough. You need to find your deeper reason for wanting to lose weight and make it known to yourself and possibly others. Write it down. Look at it. Focus on it. For example, why would a person want to lose weight to fit into their clothing? It might be so that they can look better, become confident in going out on dates, find a suitable partner, get married, and have children—their real reason is they want to have children.

Wanting children is a much more motivating goal than losing weight.

Similarly, an individual may want to lose weight to become energetic and capable of doing more things, like participating in their favorite activities, taking care of their elderly parents, babysitting, or caring for their grandchildren. It is crucial to understand that the real goal is not losing weight, and until you find your real goal, you'll likely have minimal success. Most people need help finding their actual goal, so I've included a worksheet at the back of this book to help you get started.

A great coach can help you find a deep goal or your "why." This usually takes an experienced coach who is comfortable having a personal conversation. Doing this has been relatively easy for me since I spent fourteen years working as a psychiatric RN, but getting people to go through this process when they first meet you in the gym lobby can be tough. In the gym, we aim to help people reach a deeper goal as they get to know us better.

So, when we ask, "Why is it important to lose twenty pounds?" we can eventually get to, "My blood pressure and heart health are getting to the point where I might have a heart attack if I don't change, and I don't want to leave my family without my support." That is a great goal.

Frequently, when someone starts going to the gym, their primary goal is to become healthier and more physically fit. However, many individuals may have yet to put much thought into why they want to achieve these goals, and they may have yet to share their aspirations with anyone. Here is an example of how a skilled coach might converse with someone in this situation:

The coach starts by asking why the client needs to become healthier and more physically fit, and he may answer, "I'm not healthy anymore, I'm struggling at home with some stuff, and I can't keep up with my kids anymore."

The coach then asks why it is important for him to keep up with his kids. "Because my kids are getting older, and I want to be able to do things with them."

The coach then asks why it's important to do things with his kids. "My dad was never able to do anything with me as a child; I want to be able to do things for my kids."

The coach asks again why that is important. "I want to be a good dad."

So we have a dad coming into the gym with the stated goal of getting healthier and more fit, and we end up with a goal of "I want to be a good dad." One is superficial, and one is powerful. By asking follow-up questions, we keep digging down until we help people identify a solid goal. This process takes work. A lot of coaches struggle with it; find a coach who doesn't.

Do It for Someone Else

Another way to find your real "why" or deep goal is to find a goal that focuses on someone else. Many of us will do a lot more for others than ourselves.

Wanting to feel confident about your body is a common and somewhat deep goal to lose weight. It's deeper than just wanting to lose twenty pounds because that is what you weighed in high school—but it needs to be even deeper for real motivation. If you can connect your goal with someone in your life, you have a greater chance of success. I practice this technique in my gym because I've seen that many people are not consistent in their fitness and health when their goals are about them; however, being able to take care of their mom, kids, or significant other is a much better source of motivation for their fitness and health.

Put Something on the Calendar

Events or timelines can also motivate people to reach their goals consistently. For example, I have witnessed people who want to lose a certain amount of weight to be qualified for the military do very well because the clock is ticking. Athletes who have seasons or races scheduled also have very real and in-your-face motivation. These provide straightforward and real goals to identify. For this reason, always having an event on your calendar is a good way to keep fitness first. This must be purposeful, active thought on your part. If you are asking, "What's next?" your wagon is empty. Keep that wagon full, and keep pulling it.

As a winter fat bike cyclist, if I'm not in shape, I risk freezing to death, not being able to finish, and being unable to help the people I ride with. This one race is much more motivational for me than "losing twenty pounds" or "wanting to get stronger." Keeping this race on my schedule motivates me for most of the year.

As I write this book, I recall having one of my most significant breakthroughs when I had a coach, and we did a version of the "Why Worksheet" included at the back of this book. I got to my real reason through that worksheet, but only after the coach looked at it and told me it needed to be deeper. He said, "That's not good enough. Do it again." I redid it and discovered my real "why." I didn't know what it was until that moment. I was forty-two, and no one had yet pushed me past a superficial response. Without a coach who was willing to push me, I still wouldn't know. Coaching is powerful, and great coaches are priceless.

Here are some of the most powerful hidden goals I've discovered in people using the above process. Interestingly, almost all of these people first said they came in to lose weight:

- ▶ "My husband is in a wheelchair; I need to stay strong so I can keep him in our home. He doesn't want to go to a nursing home."

- ▶ "I haven't had sex with my husband in three years because I am so uncomfortable with my body; I need to feel confident again, or he is going to leave me."

- ▶ "My wife is going to divorce me if I don't make a change; I need to start taking my health seriously."

- ▶ "Someone broke into our house while we were on vacation; if we had been home, I could not have done anything to protect my family. I need to be able to protect my family."

► "I want to outlive my wife so she doesn't have to suffer through my death."

Those are some powerful, motivational goals. Goals with emotional connection and attachment, especially to your family and loved ones, are deep. These goals lead to prolonged success in putting fitness first.

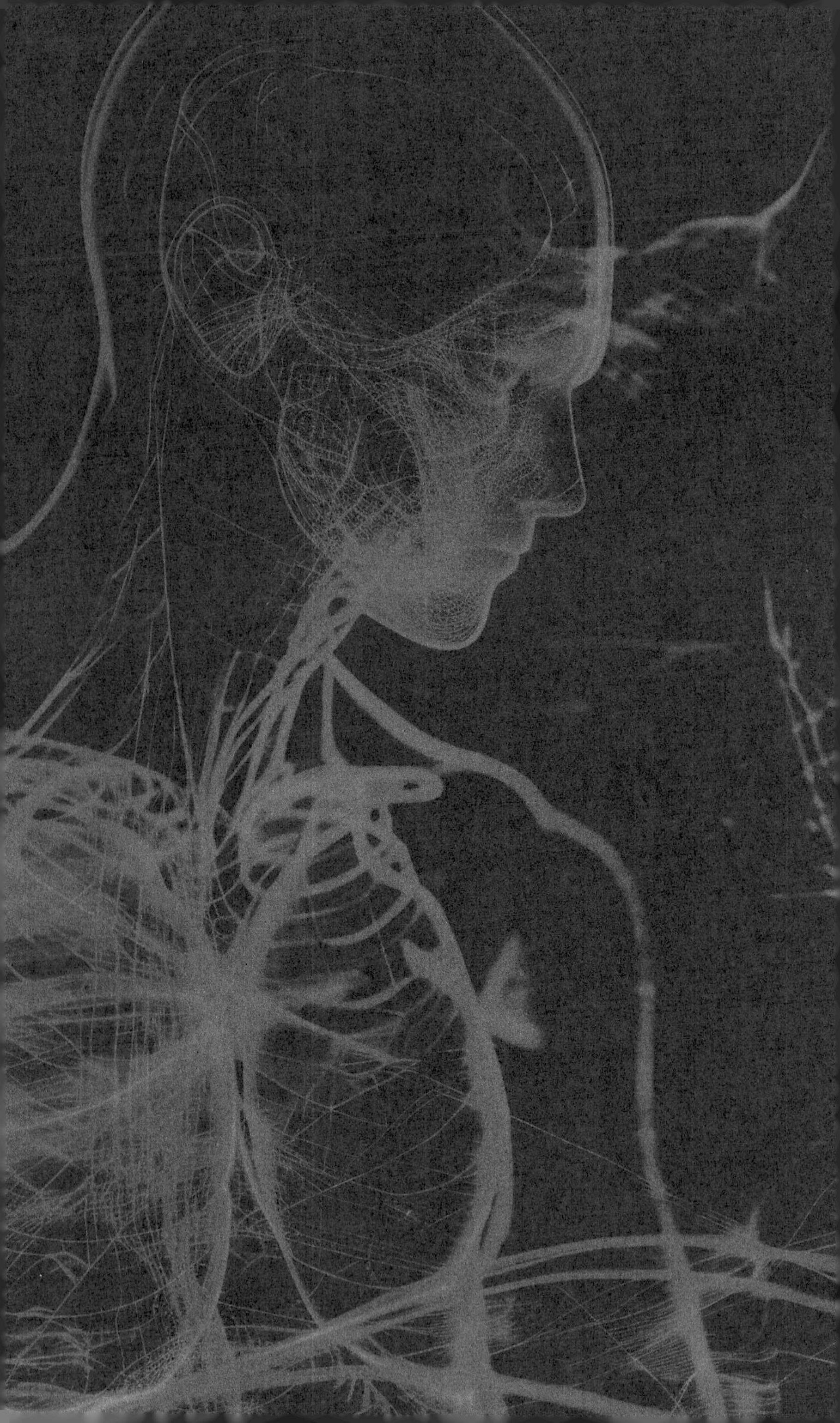

PART II

THE JOURNEY BEGINS

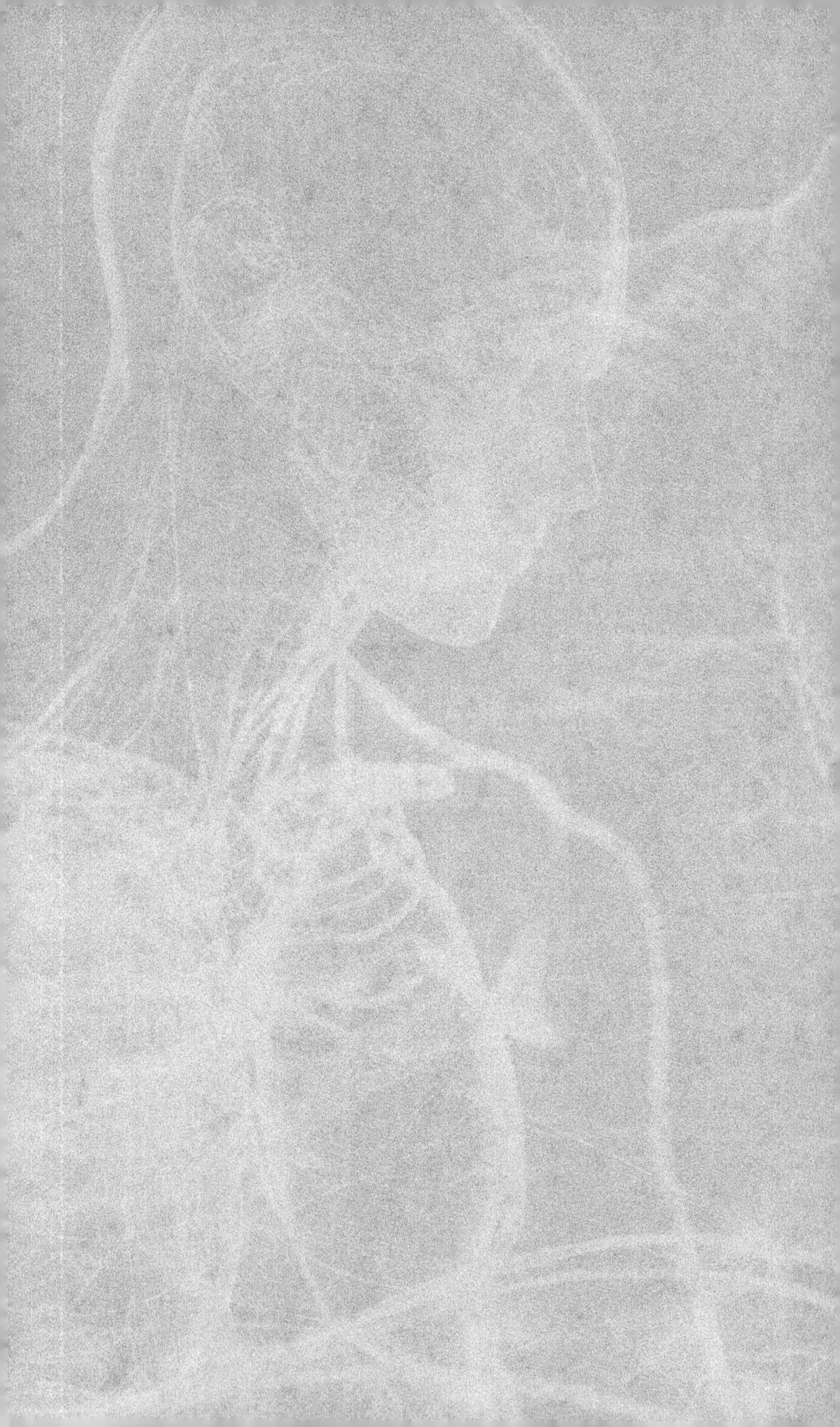

CHAPTER 5

TAKING THE FIRST STEP

Have you ever felt like you've bitten off more than you can chew, especially regarding fitness? I know I have. Let's dive into a story about a hyperactive kid (yours truly) who couldn't sit still turning into an adult and trying to figure out the fitness and health puzzle.

Back in the day, I was all over the place. My summers were spent running around like there was no tomorrow, shooting hoops, and playing all the sports. High school was no different: If a ball was involved, count me in. Then came college: I lifted weights occasionally and played basketball for fun.

Post-college, I hit the YMCA hard, playing basketball every chance I got. But my knees paid the price, so I stopped playing. The next thing I knew, I was packing on the pounds and feeling like a shadow of my former self. My health was taking a hit. My health markers started to tank, and I knew I had to get going again.

Enter CrossFit. I discovered it one night shift while dreaming of looking as ripped as the Spartans in *300*. We've all been there, right? My buddy Roo Yori and I dove headfirst into the CrossFit world, not knowing our snatches from cleans—two different weightlifting techniques—but loving every minute of it. Nine months of what we thought was CrossFit got me in the best shape of my life. It was amazing.

Deciding I was pretty good at this, I got myself a Level 1 certification in CrossFit. This was a reality check but in the best possible way. I learned how to do the movements correctly and why they worked so well, and my fitness and health data improved even more.

But why stop there? So, I dipped my toes into endurance sports like cycling, running, and triathlon, even doing this insane winter bike race that lasted up to fourteen hours. And yes, I also became "that guy" with the kettlebells because I like to keep my grip strong and my shoulders ready for anything.

Now, let's talk about starting your fitness journey. It's not about going from zero to hero overnight. It's about knowing where you are and taking it from there. If you have a history of being active, you're one step ahead. Starting from scratch? No sweat; we all start somewhere. The key is consistency—and maybe a rowing machine or a kettlebell, because who doesn't love a full-body workout with minimal equipment and investment?

Remember, starting slow and keeping at it beats going hard and burning out. And if you're new to the game, find a place that teaches you how to move well, not just how to move a lot. Trust me, your body will thank you.

If you are new to fitness, go to a functional fitness facility with a coach who knows the intricacies of movements. A coach can help you start moving your body and muscles correctly. I rarely recommend boot camp gyms for beginners; although they can be successful, the primary focus of many of those gyms is calorie burn and time spent moving. A functional fitness facility like a CrossFit gym is better for most people. Learning how to move correctly is crucial to consistency.

Surprisingly, there is still a lot of stigma around CrossFit gyms. Yet, CrossFit coaches are some of the best people I have seen teaching correct movement.

Hiring a knowledgeable coach is best if you are new to fitness or getting back into shape after a long break, but I know that is not always an option for everyone. Fortunately, there are tons of resources now. I have seen YouTube videos that are great at teaching exercise movements.

Walking!

Walking is the unsung hero of the fitness world. It's not the kind of workout that will set your Instagram on fire or rake in the likes, but we're built to walk. It's safe and effective, and you don't need to be an expert or have fancy gear to get started.

Now, walking may seem a bit ... pedestrian to some, but hear me out. Walking packs a serious fitness punch. Take it from me and my wife. We used to hit the pavement for a thirty-minute stroll every evening. Not only was it our chance to decompress and chat about our day, but it also did wonders for our fitness. A few months in, I hit the basketball court and was blown away by how much my stamina had improved. Gone were the days of gasping for air five minutes in and nursing sore muscles for what felt like an eternity after—all just from walking.

Walking is also a stealthy weapon in the battle against the bulge, particularly for folks who are new to exercise or getting back into it after a hiatus. Slipping a thirty-minute walk into your daily routine can shred pounds without you even realizing it. Swapping out the post-dinner snack for a post-dinner walk is a game-changer for your health and waistline.

So, before you reach for dessert, why not lace up and log some steps instead? Rack up those walking wins; when you're ready to kick things up a notch, venture into the world of weight training. Trust me, your body will thank you for it.

Add Weight: Resistance Training

Our bodies are begging for a bit of weight to be thrown their way. It's like they're saying, "Challenge me, and I'll reward you with muscles." And it's true; applying a bit of pressure (literally) helps us get stronger. On the flip side, if we don't, we're not doing ourselves any favors.

Resistance training isn't rocket science, but you'd be surprised how many folks don't get it quite right. It often boils down to needing to learn how. This is where the pros at functional fitness gyms, like CrossFit, come into play. They're like the Jedi masters teaching the everyday Joe and Jane how to lift, squat, and press properly.

If you don't have one of these gyms nearby, a personal trainer well-versed in basic strength training is your next best bet. This might be a tad pricier than a gym membership, but think of it as investing in not turning yourself into a pretzel while trying to deadlift. You want someone who will show you the ropes of deadlifting, back squatting, and bench pressing the right way—with actual barbells, not just moving pins on a machine. Those pin-moving machines are there so any eighteen-year-old who can say "bro" can be a personal trainer. Find a trainer who focuses on you as the machine. Splurging a bit for quality instruction is a solid investment in your health, and having a personal trainer might be the nudge you need to consistently hit your fitness goals.

Of course, there are those lone wolves who manage just fine solo. If that's you, more power to you. First, just spend some time (and maybe a few bucks) learning the correct techniques. Stick with the basics, nail them, and only then, think about getting fancy. The key here is consistency and mastering the fundamentals before showing off the fancy stuff.

Get Your Heart Going: Cardio

Cardio—that term we all love to hate—is about getting your heart to beat faster than its normal, everyday pace. It's essential for shedding pounds and maintaining a healthy heart, not to mention preparing it for when it needs to work overtime.

Kicking off your cardio journey might seem like a puzzle, but it's not a 1,000-piece puzzle. Let's break it down into simple steps to help you weave some heart-pumping action into your routine. I'll focus on jogging here because it's the most accessible form of cardio—all you need are shoes:

► **STEP 1:** Begin with easy jogs. Think about jogging around your local area or park for one to twenty minutes. Not a fan of the great outdoors? Then, treadmills are your friend.

► **STEP 2:** Remember to take it easy. Short breaks are your allies, not enemies. Are you feeling winded or just not up for it? Walking is totally fine. Slow and steady wins the race, and consistency beats going all out right from the get-go. Jogging for thirty seconds and walking for sixty seconds will still benefit your health.

► **STEP 3:** As you start feeling more like the Duracell bunny and less like a sloth, crank up the duration and distance of your jogs. Try alternating between two minutes of jogging and two minutes of walking. When that feels like a walk in the park, bump up your jog time by a minute while keeping your walking breaks the same length. Keep upping your game until walking breaks feel like an option rather than a necessity.

The same process above can be applied to using cardio equipment. Remember, starting slow and being consistent wins over going out hard and quitting.

Once you've mastered walking, lifting, and cardio, it's time to dial up the intensity. Let's get that heart racing and those muscles burning!

Go Harder: Intensity

Intensity can turbocharge your weight loss and fitness goals in a fraction of the time. Like any powerful remedy, intensity is the closest thing to a fitness miracle cure; however, it comes with its caveats—mainly, the risks of injury and burnout.

Injuries often happen when folks jump into high gear with movements they're not used to. Cranking up the intensity without having the basics down is like trying to run before you can walk–literally and figuratively. Fitness is a marathon, not a sprint. If you're new to exercise, remember that any form of movement is beneficial. There's no need to push into the red zone right away. Use the initial phase to get your movements right. Then, when you're ready to turn up the dial, your body will be prepped for it.

This is another area where a good coach comes into play. A keen eye can prevent you from pushing too hard too soon and ending up on the sidelines. A great coach doesn't just play defense; they'll know exactly when you're ready to accelerate.

When safely adding intensity, machines like air bikes are your best bet. They let you go all out with a much lower risk of injury. Air bikes are pretty straightforward, making them a solid choice for feeling the burn safely. Rowing machines are another fantastic option, though they require more technique. Investing time with a coach to nail down the proper rowing form can make all the difference.

Intensity has its place in a well-rounded fitness regimen. The key is to approach it thoughtfully, building up to it in a way that safeguards your well-being.

If you've ticked off all the boxes and are looking for the next challenge, channeling your fitness into sports is a fantastic way to keep your body and mind in shape.

Play Sports

Diving into sports is like hitting the jackpot of physical activity. With the sheer variety out there, something will catch your eye—whether it's the adrenaline rush of intense cardio, the power surge from lifting, or the zen focus of hitting that perfect shot. The cool part is they all get you moving and motivated. Who doesn't love the thrill of getting better at something they enjoy?

Sports also add a social element to the mix. Joining a team or casual group has a way of bringing people together like nothing else. You're all sweating it out, chasing the same goal, and building camaraderie. Sports create bonds that can last a lifetime and foster a sense of community that goes beyond the game. And as we all know, how you treat your body off the field or court makes a huge difference in how you perform during the game; neglect your health, and it's going to show.

Picking up a sport you used to love or finding a new one to dive into is easier than you think. Maybe there's a game you aced as a kid that you've been itching to get back into? Just remember to pace yourself. There are better ways to go than rushing in and ending up injured. Start slow; get those muscles and joints used to moving again.

And if the sport of your glory days isn't in the cards anymore or if you've never really been the sporting type, the world's your oyster. There's a wealth of activities out there waiting for you to take a swing at them. Have you ever thought about giving golf or disc golf a go? How about pickleball? These are excellent options for those looking to blend activity with skill sharpening.

The bottom line? It doesn't matter what sport or activity you choose. The key is to get moving. Considering how much of our days are spent sitting, introducing more movement into our lives is essential. Start with walking, and then graduate to something that gets your heart racing a bit more. Fitness is a journey with one fantastic destination: a healthier you.

As we transition into the next chapter, the focus shifts to consistency in your fitness journey. Consistency is the glue that holds your fitness together, transforming sporadic efforts into lasting habits and tangible results. It's about starting strong, maintaining momentum, adapting to challenges, and finding joy.

The upcoming section will explore strategies for staying committed to your fitness goals, overcoming obstacles, and integrating exercise into your daily life as a nonnegotiable part of your routine, including insights on making fitness a consistent, rewarding part of your life journey.

CONSISTENCY: YOUR PATH TO SUCCESS

Sticking to a new health and fitness routine can be challenging. Prioritizing a fitness routine and mindset is difficult but not impossible among your daily life tasks. Several studies have found valuable practices and strategies for maintaining consistency and motivation to succeed in your fitness journey. Below are some key insights based on the latest research:

- ► **SET REALISTIC GOALS:** Your starting point should be building achievable and specific goals. Overly ambitious goals can lead to disappointment and dropout, so gradual progression is more sustainable and reachable.

- ► **CREATE A ROUTINE:** Consistency is a magic pill in your fitness journey. Schedule your workouts like any other important activity. A routine helps establish exercise as a habit.

► **FIND ACTIVITIES YOU ENJOY:** If you enjoy the activities, you may be more likely to stick with a routine. Experiment with different types of exercise to find what you like.

► **TRACK YOUR PROGRESS:** Recording your workouts and progress can motivate your journey. It allows you to see improvements over time and helps you set targets.

► **SOCIAL SUPPORT:** Getting engaged with a community, whether it is a fitness class, online community, or a workout buddy, can increase accountability and make exercise more enjoyable.

► **REWARD YOURSELF:** Set up a system of rewards for reaching your fitness goals. It can provide additional push and a sense of achievement.

► **MINDSET AND SELF-COMPASSION:** It is crucial to adopt a positive mindset toward fitness and be compassionate when facing obstacles in your journey. Always remember that it is okay to miss a workout, but what's important is getting back on track.

► **SMART USE OF TECHNOLOGY:** Fitness trackers, apps, and online resources can provide structure, guidance, and additional motivation.

► **FOCUS ON HEALTH, NOT JUST APPEARANCE:** Focusing on the health benefits of exercise, like improved mood, better sleep, and increased energy, can be more motivating than focusing solely on appearance-based goals.

► **INCREASE INTENSITY:** To avoid burnout and injury, gradually increase your workout's intensity level and duration.

► **CONNECT TO YOUR BODY:** Pay attention to your body's signals. Rest and recovery are essential parts of every fitness journey.

► **CONSULT PROFESSIONALS:** For personalized advice and to ensure you are on the right track, consider consulting fitness and health professionals. An expert will help you get started and increase your chances of developing a consistent habit.

Research in behavioral psychology suggests that understanding your barriers to exercise and actively planning for them—for example, scheduling workouts for when you are least likely to cancel–can significantly improve adherence to a fitness routine.

The key to sticking with a health and fitness routine is finding what works for you. Individual preferences and lifestyles significantly influence what is sustainable and enjoyable. Here are some examples of how these strategies have helped many people in my gyms stay consistent for long periods:

- ► Keep track of workouts on a calendar. "Even if I was working and driving daily from the cities, they stayed on my calendar. My assistant also knew how to schedule my workouts."

- ► Have an accountability partner at the gym. "Having someone ask, 'Where were you yesterday?!' is powerful motivation."

- ► Do not get out of the habit. "I only allowed a few days to go by without a workout, even at home or traveling. Because once you let go of it, it becomes hard to get back on it."

- ► Set timely goals and revisit them frequently. "You don't have to do a weight loss diet or lift weights together. You can do one at a time. One of my most important goals every year is just to be able to keep playing with my grandchildren."

► Enjoy the feeling working out gives you. "Once your workouts become routine, you will not feel good when you miss them. Interestingly, that habit also keeps you going."

Putting It into Action

Setting and prioritizing your routine before the day starts goes a long way and can help you create a consistent fitness routine. Here are some strategies that I have seen work best over the years.

Morning Workouts

The easiest way to find time to exercise is to get up earlier. Almost everyone can employ this strategy. People who are committed to this habit achieve great success in their lives, waking up at 4 a.m. and heading to the gym or basement for a workout.

You may think, "I am not a morning person," "I can't get up that early," or "I am a night owl," but these feelings are not unique. There are very few "natural" morning people. Morning people are made, not born.

Your next step should be to arrange your evening so you can go to bed earlier. Your will-power will get you out of bed for a few days, but it will not get you out of bed for weeks, months, and years. For many people with kids, the later evening time is their "me time," so it's critical to shift your mentality to having that "me time" in the early morning. For many people, this change is enough.

Noon Workouts

After early morning workouts, working out during lunch is also an option if your job allows it. Lunch-hour workouts are a great way to get into a routine that's built into your workday. People who work out around noon have great success with consistency and results because friends or co-workers often surround them while they work out.

This is an added form of accountability and motivation. Co-workers who work out together can become a powerful force. Research also shows that people who work out during the day are mentally sharper and display better teamwork.

Evening Workouts

If early morning workouts or the noon hour doesn't work for you, then after work is also an excellent option. Evening workouts can become a celebration of the end of the workday, but some people have difficulty with them because that time is often full of other familial duties. Look at your daily schedule and see what time will be the easiest to implement into your routine.

Don't Burn Yourself Out.

Remember to take it easy. Go slow. Save some for tomorrow. The most common mistake people who are new to fitness make is going too hard. It is one of the reasons I encourage walking and not running for beginners or starting with a personal trainer instead of joining a gym. Doing a workout designed to crush your soul on day one is generally a terrible idea; this path will make you so sore and worthless for the next few days that you decide not to go back to the gym for a week.

Get a Coach, and Have a Plan

When starting on your fitness path, having a coach helps tremendously. Find an expert with a history of success. Sorry, but this isn't going to be the kid at the local 24/7 gym. A great coach will be able to help you in all areas: finding your goals, starting you on the right program, and getting you through the times you want to quit.

Goals Are Key

As discussed in chapter four, I've found that goals tied to other people or nonphysical attributes have more sticking power than the usual goals you will set when starting at the gym. The years I have spent in the gym have proven over and over again that a weight loss goal that's not tied to something else rarely works long-term. Long-term success increases if you connect it to health, family, or a loved one.

Your success is tied to you finding a reason worth working for, and that reason may change over time. You must dig deep when setting your goals, so consistency becomes a byproduct of your internal drive. It will become hard not to exercise; instead of skipping workouts, you may skip rest days. Allow yourself to fall in love with the process, and over time, consistency will get you to your goals.

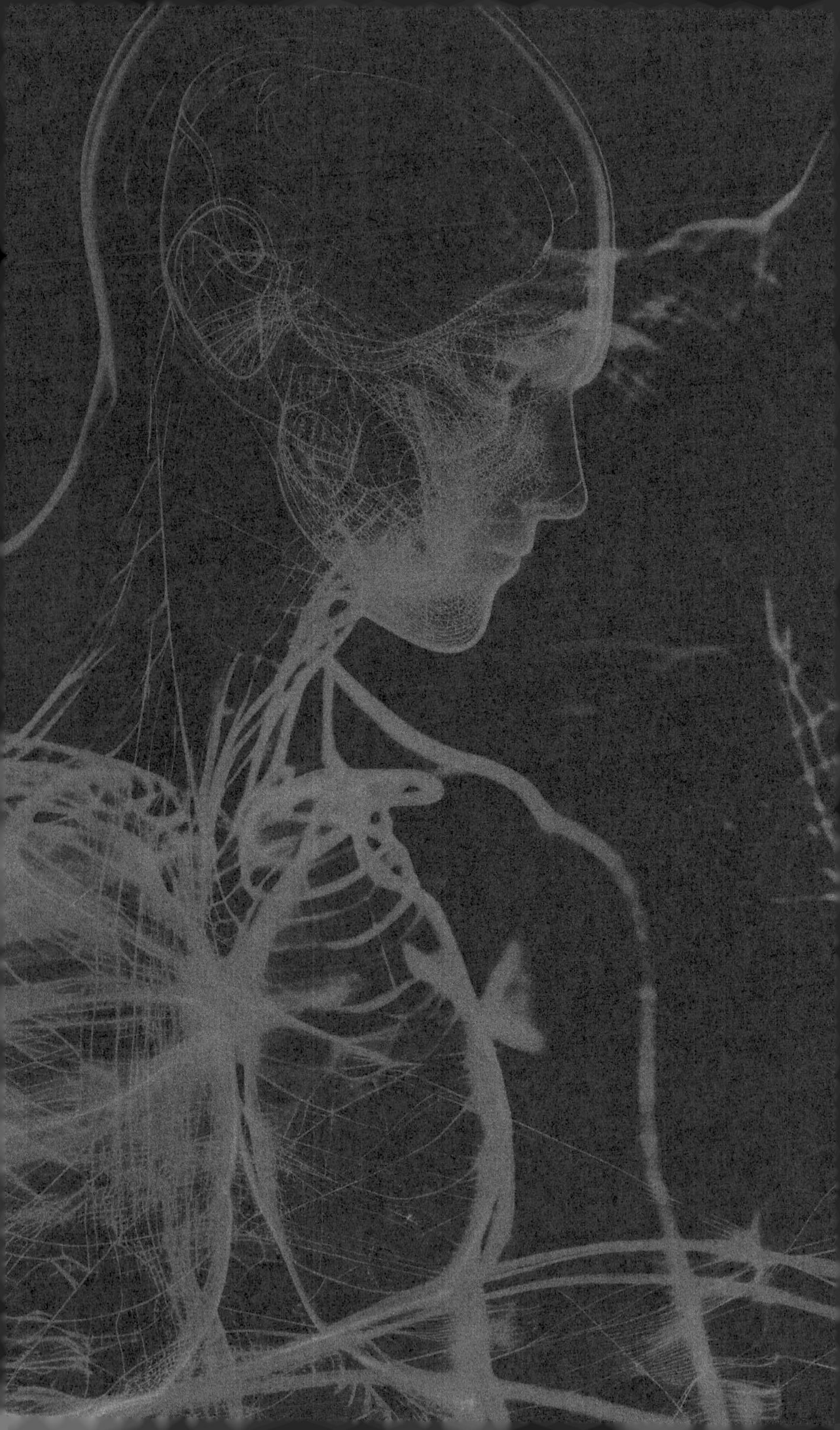

PART III

BUILDING THE FOUNDATION

CHAPTER 7

THE POWER OF COMMUNITY

The Köhler Effect

Have you ever noticed that you just kill it in a group workout, pushing past what you thought were your limits? That is the Köhler effect in action: We find ourselves stepping up our game in a team setting, especially when we think we might be the underdogs.

No one wants to be the weak link. When the success of our group hangs in the balance, and it seems like we're the ones everyone's waiting on, we dig deep and find that extra gear, pushing harder than we ever do solo. It's all about not wanting to let the team down.

This isn't just about a one-time burst of effort either. The Köhler effect means we're also more likely to keep at it session after session because we're fueled by the energy of not wanting to drop the ball for our team. Before I knew this phenomenon had a name, I wrote a blog post about it, called "Chasing Rabbits." In short, it stated that you need to be around people working hard to improve, and for others to improve, you must also work hard.

The Köhler effect is a large part of why fitness communities or group challenges can be so effective. It taps into our social wiring, pushing us to not only meet our personal goals but also contribute to a collective victory. We're driven to prove to ourselves and others that we've got what it takes, especially when we're all in it together.

The downside of the Köhler effect is that it can make people work harder than they are physically prepared to work, so if a CrossFit gym wants you to do some personal training before throwing you into group classes, this is one reason why.

Community is about more than performance.

A supportive community is pivotal in maintaining fitness habits. Its power cannot be underestimated; it helps foster a commitment to fitness, while promoting the overall well-being of its members.

In addition to increasing performance, it boosts motivation and enhances emotional health, including a reduction in stress and anxiety—which are often barriers to maintaining a consistent exercise routine.

Community Accountability

An accountability buddy can significantly contribute to you reaching your fitness goals. When you have someone to keep you in check, you are more likely to stick to your workout routine and make healthier choices.

This can lead to more consistent exercise habits and better overall fitness outcomes. For example, if a friend is counting on you to show up at the gym at 5 a.m., you are less likely to hit the snooze button and skip your workout. This kind of accountability can provide the extra push you need to stay committed to your fitness journey, especially on challenging days when motivation is low.

Finding a Community

When it comes to finding a community, you can employ several strategies. Joining a gym is probably the easiest way. I have met a few "frequent movers" who have told me the first thing they do when they get to a new town is find a CrossFit gym: "I have 100 new friends in a week."

If you think gyms are not for you, try a few more. Every gym is different. If your choices are slim, online communities can be effective for some. Platforms like Instagram and Facebook are filled with fitness enthusiasts who share their journeys, tips, and challenges, creating an online space for individuals to find inspiration and support.

It's important to acknowledge that finding the right fitness community takes time. It's okay to explore different options and "date around" to find the perfect match. Each fitness community has unique dynamics, and you should seek an environment that aligns with your fitness goals, values, and preferences.

The role of a community in empowering you to reach your fitness goals cannot be overlooked. From the Köhler effect to reduced stress and anxiety, it may be the missing piece of the puzzle if you have not succeeded in your fitness journey and have not yet tried a community-based approach.

CHAPTER 8

CULTIVATING A FITNESS MINDSET

Past success is usually the best predictor of future success. Have you completed long-term projects or tasks in the past? If so, then there's a good chance you'll do so again. I have worked for managers who hired employees simply because they had a four-year degree. They don't even care what that person studied; the degree proves they could complete a long-term task. They have demonstrated past success—and an expensive demonstration at that.

Of course, success does not necessarily translate into getting out of bed at five a.m. to exert yourself physically. These are different beasts. People who are very successful in one area are not always successful in another: for example, the super fit guy who works in a dead-end job well below his potential, or on the other end of the spectrum, the uber-successful businessman who is obese and on his way to an early grave.

But individuals can often use success in one area to gain success in another. Confidence and a history of success go a long way in getting things done, even if the new thing is different and challenging.

Suppose you have no history of success in health and fitness. In that case, the first step is spending time identifying areas in your life that you are successful in. If you can't think of any, ask other people. In the unlikely event you still can't think of anything, make finishing this book your first goal toward a life of accomplishment.

Mind Tricks and Micro-Decisions

The difference between success and failure almost always comes down to mental tools, and fortunately, these can be learned and improved.

The success or failure of any endeavor is determined by a series of small decisions that we make every day, which are known as micro-decisions. Our mindset influences these micro-decisions. Negative thoughts like "I can't do this," "I won't be able to do this for long," or "I've never been able to do this before" can hold us back from achieving our goals.

Suppose we believe that we're genetically programmed to be overweight. In that case, we are more likely to fail in our weight loss efforts. Likewise, if we approach our task with the idea that we can only stick to a diet for seven days before having a cheat day, we are setting ourselves up for failure.

To succeed, we must reject these negative thoughts and beliefs early on. As the saying goes, "If you think you can't, you're right." This applies to most aspects of our lives, including our ability to make good micro-decisions.

Mind tricks are ways of reframing your thinking to cope with difficult situations. They differ from person to person, meaning what works for one might not work for another. Some of these tricks may seem strange, but they can be very effective. The key is to find the one that works best for you. Here are a few examples:

- ► When I worked in a nursing unit, there were tasty treats in the nursing conference room every week. This made it difficult for those on a meal plan to resist the temptation of sugar. To combat this, I imagined the donuts covered in poop. I've worked in healthcare for over twenty years and have seen my fair share of poop, so it wasn't hard for me to visualize. I even joked with my coworkers about it. This technique helped me resist the treats, even though they were right in front of me most days of the week.

► One trick I will have some people use during an exercise is to picture their child or someone important to them at the finish line. There are various levels of this trick ranging from just getting to your child for a hug to getting to them in time because they need your help.

► For some people, looking at their body as an experiment or a playfield can be an effective way to get to certain goals or milestones. This is often called the "let's see what happens" or "let's try an experiment" game. It involves thoughts like "I am just going to try this to see what happens" or "This is just a trial. I am not committing to anything, just testing." This can help reduce the hesitation of starting a new program or lifestyle.

There are many other techniques I've used in different situations for myself and my clients. These tricks are not unique to me and are often used by professional athletes or those working with psychologists or performance coaches. The human mind is a powerful tool, and these techniques can help you hack it to overcome difficult situations.

The Dial Versus the Switch

Imagine that you crush a week at the gym, but by Saturday, you feel sluggish and unmotivated, so you stay home, sleep in, eat a poor breakfast, and then spend the day making poor choices all because you think you already messed up your morning. I call this all-or-nothing thinking, "flipping the switch."

But what if instead of calling the day a loss, you decided to do just a little activity instead of skipping your workout entirely. You get up, move, head to the gym, and hop on a rower with the intent to row easy for twenty minutes. After twenty minutes, you can be done, or if you are feeling better, you can keep going. I refer to this as "turning the dial." Just because you don't feel like doing a grueling, intense workout doesn't mean you can't do an easy one. Turning the dial up and down is much better than flipping the switch on and off. This is true for how strict you are on your diet, the amount you exercise, and your workout intensity.

Turning the switch off and on may get short-term changes but not long-term results or effects. With the switch mentality, you might say to yourself. "I ate a donut . . . so I may as well eat pizza. I ate some pizza, so I may have a beer. I had a beer, so I might have a couple more."

Switching to a "dial" mentality will help you reach your goals faster. Instead of the above dialogue, you'd have the following: "I had a donut. Cool. Now, I will dial myself back to where I want to be. The day is not lost." Dialing it back is not going to destroy your weeks of dedicated consistency, but a weekend with the switch off might. Not doing anything on Thursday could turn into nothing on Friday, leading to nothing on Saturday, and then when Monday rolls around, you're right where you were last Monday. If you stop everything you're doing, you are going to backslide.

Setting Goals the Right Way

Setting clear fitness goals is essential for several reasons. First, it provides direction and purpose to your fitness journey. Without specific goals, it's easy to lose focus and motivation. In chapter three, we discussed the importance of finding a powerful "why." Goals ensure we get to and can accomplish our "why," and they also offer a way to measure progress, helping track achievements and identify improvement areas.

SMART Goals in Fitness

A helpful framework for setting practical fitness goals is the SMART acronym:

- ► **SPECIFIC:** Goals should be clear and specific. Instead of setting a vague goal like "get fit," specify what "fit" means. This could be running a certain distance, lifting a specific weight, or achieving a particular body composition.

- ► **MEASURABLE:** Your goals should be quantifiable. This makes it possible to track progress. For instance, rather than aiming to "lose weight," set a goal to lose a certain number of pounds or kilograms.

- ► **ACHIEVABLE:** While goals should be challenging, they must also be realistic and attainable. Setting an unrealistic goal can lead to disappointment and demotivation.

- **RELEVANT:** Your fitness goals should relate to your desires, interests, lifestyle, and your "why." Goals that align with your values and life situation are more motivating.

- **TIME-BOUND:** Assign a timeframe to your goals. Having a deadline creates a sense of urgency and can spur action.

SMART goals get a lot of flack in the media; however, they work very well when done correctly. In my years of helping people set goals in the hospital setting and the gym, I've found that the first try at setting a SMART goal is rarely done correctly. Even with clear directions, most people need assistance seeing the errors in their SMART goal formula.

Examples of strong fitness SMART goals include:

- I want to run a 5K in under thirty minutes within the next three months.

- I want to attend yoga classes twice a week for the next six months.

- I want to increase my strength to deadlift 150 pounds within the next four months.

I ran goal-setting groups for fourteen years in the hospital setting and can assert that clear SMART goals, like the examples above, are effective. Once SMART goals are in place, you then will set even more specific goals to get to these goals. This is called a roadmap.

Creating a Roadmap for Your Goals

Once your goals are set, create a roadmap for achieving them by breaking down the larger goal into smaller, more manageable tasks. For instance, if your goal is to run a 5K, start with shorter runs of a specified length, and gradually increase your distance each week by a specified amount. My clients frequently create multiple short-term goals to work toward a long-term goal. The same rules apply for creating short-term goals as for long-term goals.

Monitoring and Adjusting Goals

Review your goals regularly to track your progress. Celebrate the small victories as they contribute to the more significant achievement. Be flexible and willing to adjust your goals if circumstances change or if they are too easy or challenging.

Setting clear goals lays a strong foundation for a successful fitness journey. These goals act as a compass, guiding your efforts and keeping you focused on what's important.

Overcoming Mental Barriers

Mental barriers, such as fear of failure, lack of confidence, or procrastination, often stall fitness progress. Identifying and addressing these barriers is crucial. Techniques like journaling can help you recognize and understand these mental blocks. Once identified, setting smaller, achievable goals can then help you gradually overcome these barriers.

Mindfulness practices can also be effective in dealing with mental obstacles. Being mindful helps you stay present and not get overwhelmed by negative thoughts or future anxieties. It allows you to focus on your current abilities and efforts rather than getting bogged down by what you can't do or still need to achieve.

Cognitive Behavioral Techniques (CBT) in Fitness

Cognitive Behavioral Therapy (CBT) focuses on changing patterns of thinking or behavior behind people's difficulties and, in turn, changing how they feel. It involves recognizing distorted thinking and reframing thoughts more positively and realistically. CBT techniques can be adapted to enhance your fitness journey.

For example, if you tend to think, "I missed my workout today; I'll never be fit," CBT would encourage you to reframe this thought to "Missing one workout doesn't define my fitness journey. I can get back on track tomorrow." Or by using the "turning the dial" technique, you could go for a walk to get some activity and frame that as a win. This reframing helps maintain a positive and resilient mindset toward fitness.

Building a Supportive Mindset

Surrounding yourself with positive influences and a supportive community can reinforce your fitness-first mentality. As we discussed in the last chapter, engaging with fitness communities, either online or in person, can provide motivation, advice, and a sense of belonging. Sharing your goals and progress with friends or a fitness coach can also provide accountability and encouragement.

Incorporating these cognitive strategies into your daily routine can significantly impact your fitness journey. They help build a resilient, positive mindset that drives you towards your fitness goals and enhances your overall quality of life.

Mindfulness and Meditation for Focus

Mindfulness and meditation are effective mental exercises for maintaining motivation in fitness. Mindfulness involves being fully present and engaged at the moment, aware of your thoughts and feelings without distraction or judgment. This practice helps you focus on your fitness activities, enhance the mind-body connection, and reduce stress, often a barrier to consistent exercise.

Meditation, particularly focused meditation, can be beneficial for fitness enthusiasts. It involves concentrating on a single focus point, such as breathing or a mantra, which can improve concentration and mental clarity. These qualities are essential for staying motivated and committed to fitness goals. I started a meditation practice during the COVID-19 pandemic. It was a tough time, and meditation immensely helped me stay focused on what I needed to do to stay healthy and provide for my family and friends.

Mental Rehearsal for Success

Mental rehearsal, or visualization of success, is a technique athletes use to enhance performance. It involves mentally practicing a physical activity or visualizing achieving a goal. For instance, before a workout, take a few minutes to close your eyes and imagine yourself completing the exercises. Visualize the movements, the environment, and the feeling of accomplishment. This mental rehearsal can boost confidence and performance during the actual activity.

Gratitude Practices in Daily Fitness

Incorporating gratitude into your fitness routine can have a positive impact on motivation. At the end of each workout, take a moment to reflect on what you are grateful for. This may be your body's ability to move, your progress, or the opportunity to be active. This practice shifts the focus from what you have to achieve to what you have already accomplished, fostering a sense of satisfaction and encouraging continued effort.

These mental exercises are about improving physical performance and cultivating a mindset that values and enjoys the fitness journey.

Practicing mindfulness, mental rehearsal, and gratitude reinforces your commitment to fitness and enhances your overall well-being.

Remember, fitness first is not just about the physical transformation; it's about cultivating a mindset that values health and well-being as fundamental components of a happy and fulfilling life. Celebrate your successes, learn from your setbacks, and always strive for progress, not perfection. Fitness is not a destination but a way of living, a continuous journey of self-improvement and self-discovery.

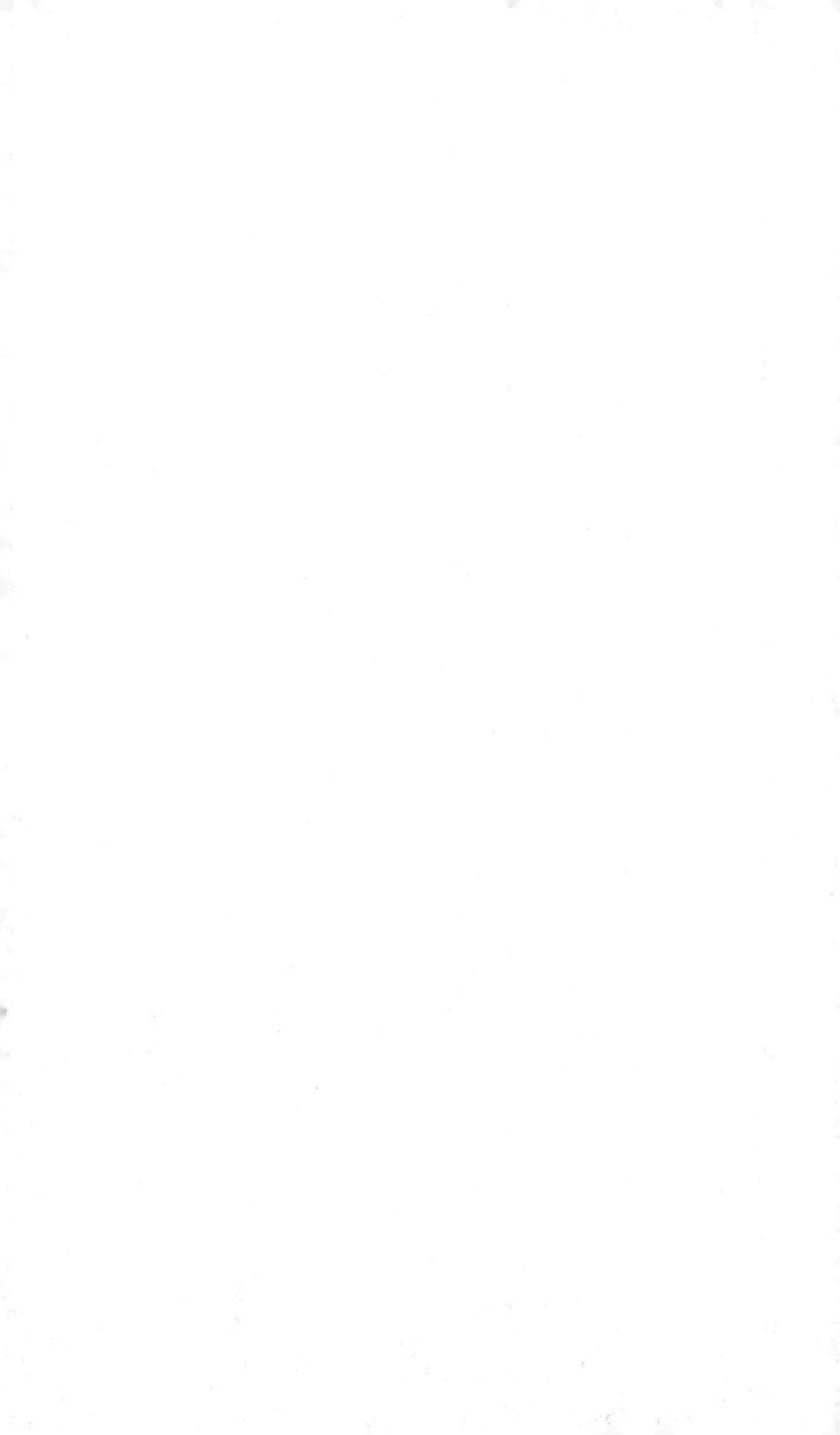

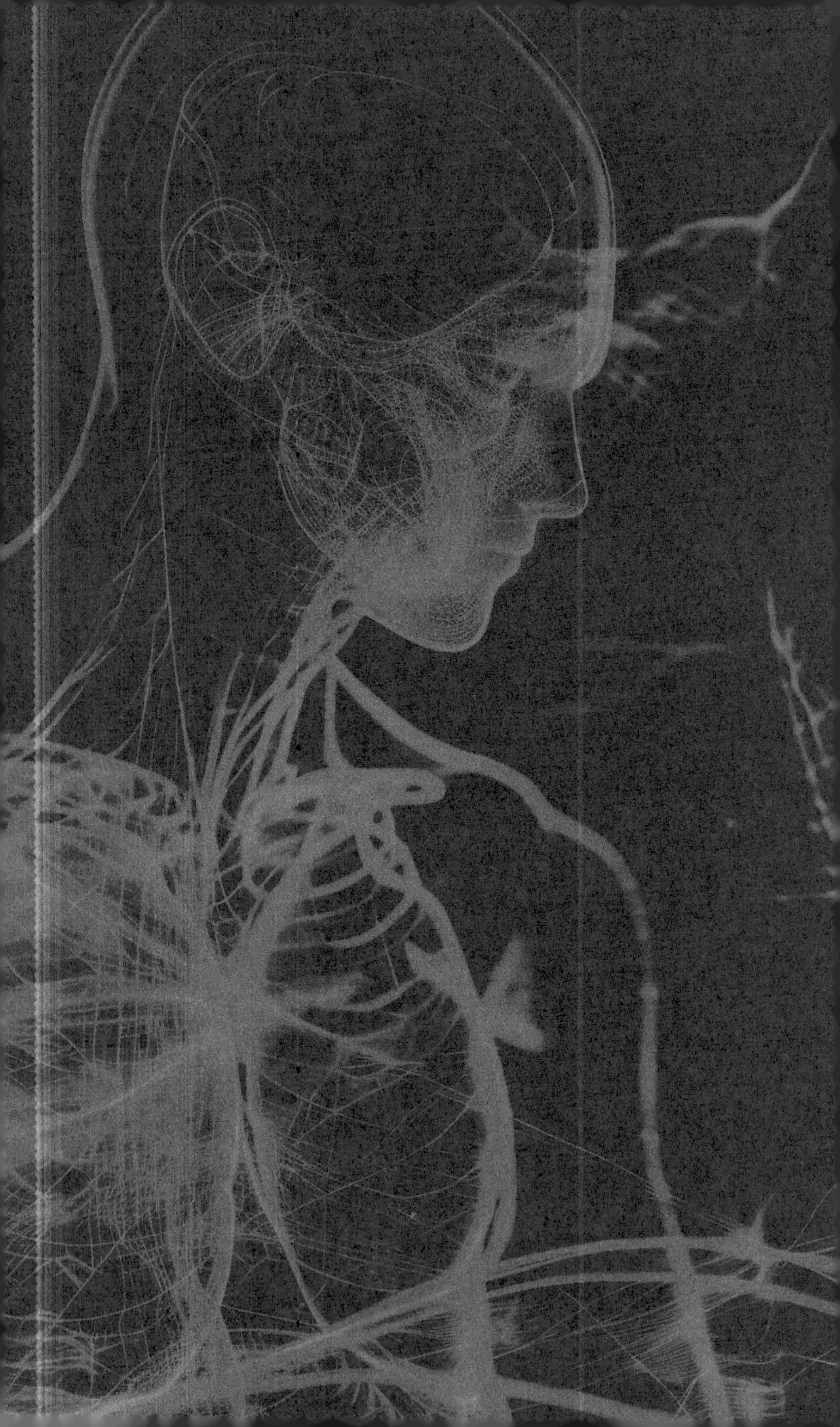

SUSTAINABLE HABITS

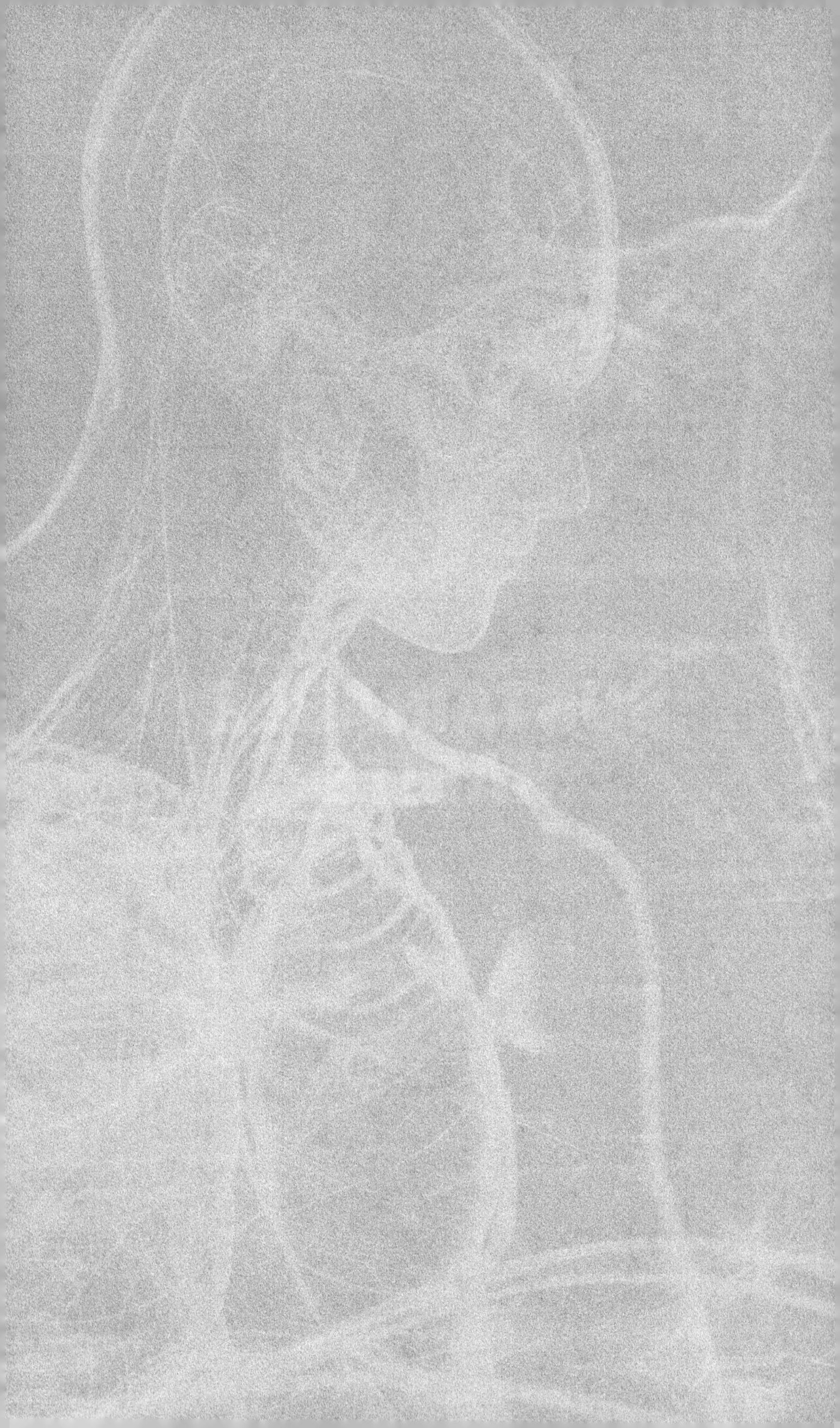

CHAPTER 9

BUILDING LASTING HABITS

Developing a fitness-first mentality is more than just incorporating a series of workouts and diet plans; it's about building sustainable habits that lead to long-term success. The key to maintaining fitness commitment lies not just in the intensity of exercises or the strictness of diets but in the seemingly small daily habits that create a foundation for a healthy lifestyle. Understanding the science behind habit formation and its impact on fitness is crucial for anyone looking to transform their physical health and well-being.

This chapter will delve into habit formation and its psychological motives and provide practical strategies for building and maintaining fitness habits. You can create a fitness routine—it just takes a little practice and persistence.

The Science Behind Habit Formation

Habit formation is a fascinating process rooted in neuroscience. Habits are our brain's way of saving effort. When a behavior becomes a habit, it transitions from an active, conscious decision to an automatic response. This shift occurs in the basal ganglia, which play a crucial role in developing emotions, memories, and pattern recognition. Simply put, initially, you need to do what will seem like hard work, but after a while, this hard work turns into autopilot and becomes easy.

Initially, when we perform a new task, our prefrontal cortex, the area responsible for decision-making and conscious thought, is highly active. However, as this behavior is repeated over time, the activity in the prefrontal cortex decreases, and the basal ganglia take over. This transition marks the behavior's evolution into a habit.

The Role of the Brain in Developing and Sustaining Habits

Neuroplasticity, the brain's ability to reorganize itself by forming new neural connections, plays a significant role in habit formation. Every time we repeat a behavior, we strengthen the neural pathways associated with it, making it easier and more natural to perform over time. This is why habits, once established, can become so ingrained that they feel automatic. It is also why if you have a fitness guru as a friend, they may tell you certain things are easy, but to you, they seem impossible.

During habit formation, the brain releases dopamine, a neurotransmitter associated with pleasure and reward. This release occurs when the habit is executed and when the brain anticipates the habitual activity. This anticipation of reward helps solidify the habit.

Understanding the neurological basis of habit formation is crucial in developing sustainable fitness habits. Recognizing that habits result from repeated behaviors and neural adaptations can provide insight into why forming new habits can be challenging, yet incredibly rewarding in the long run.

Psychological Principles Behind Habit Formation

The formation of fitness habits is deeply rooted in various psychological principles. One key concept is the "habit loop," which consists of three components: the cue (the trigger), the routine (the behavior itself), and the reward. The cue triggers the behavior, and the reward reinforces it, creating a loop that encourages the behavior to be repeated.

Another essential principle is self-efficacy: the belief in one's ability to succeed in specific situations. When it comes to fitness, believing in your ability to stick to a workout routine or maintain a healthy diet is crucial. This belief is reinforced every time you complete a workout or make a healthy food choice, gradually strengthening the habit.

How Habits Influence Long-Term Fitness Commitment

Habits play a pivotal role in long-term commitment to fitness for several reasons. Firstly, once a habit is formed, it requires less mental effort and decision-making, making it more likely to be maintained. For example, if going for a run first thing in the morning becomes habitual, it becomes an automatic part of your routine rather than something you must consciously decide to do every day.

Habits can create a ripple effect, positively influencing other areas of your life. Regular exercise, for instance, can lead to better sleep patterns, improved mood, and higher energy levels, reinforcing the exercise habit and motivating you to continue.

However, forming fitness habits isn't just about repetition; it's also about creating a positive and rewarding experience. If the rewards of fitness—whether physical, emotional, or mental—are significant and recognized, the desire to continue the habit strengthens.

Key Elements of Sustainable Fitness Habits

Consistency and Routine

Consistency is the cornerstone of sustainable habit formation. When it comes to fitness, establishing a consistent routine is crucial. This doesn't necessarily mean working out every day; it means setting a manageable schedule that aligns with your lifestyle. Consistency in your fitness routine reinforces the neural pathways associated with your exercise habits, making them stronger and more automatic over time.

Reward and Motivation

The reward component of the habit loop is essential in sustaining a fitness habit. The reward must be immediate and satisfying to reinforce the behavior. In the context of fitness, the reward can vary from the endorphin rush after a workout to the sense of achievement in reaching a milestone. Recognizing and celebrating these rewards is important, as they are vital motivators in maintaining the habit.

Cue-Routine-Reward Cycle in Fitness

Understanding and effectively utilizing the cue-routine-reward cycle is vital in building fitness habits. A cue can be a specific time of the day, a particular location, a preceding event, or even an emotional state. For example, laying out your workout clothes the night before can be a visual cue to exercise in the morning. The routine is the workout itself, and the reward could be a sense of accomplishment or a healthy post-workout snack.

Successfully integrating this cycle into your daily life involves identifying the right cues that prompt your fitness routines and ensuring the rewards are meaningful and satisfying. When repeated, this cycle forms the basis of a strong fitness habit.

Flexibility within Habits

While consistency is vital, flexibility within your fitness habits is also essential. Life is unpredictable, and being too rigid with your habits can lead to frustration and burnout. Allowing flexibility in your routine, such as changing your workout type or timing on hectic days, can help you maintain the habit without feeling overwhelmed.

Strategies for Building Fitness Habits

Practical Techniques Based on Psychological Principles:

- ▶ **START SMALL AND GRADUALLY INCREASE DIFFICULTY:** Begin with small, manageable fitness activities and gradually increase the intensity or duration. This aligns with the psychological principle of shaping, where behaviors are developed by gradually reinforcing closer approximations to the desired behavior. For instance, start with a ten-minute walk each day, and slowly increase it to a thirty-minute jog.

- ▶ **USE HABIT STACKING:** This strategy involves stacking a new habit onto an existing one. This leverages the principle of association, making it easier to adopt the new habit. For example, if you have an established habit of drinking coffee every morning, stack a five-minute stretching routine right before or after this existing habit.

Incorporating Habits into Different Lifestyles:

► **CUSTOMIZE YOUR FITNESS ROUTINE:** Adapting your fitness habits to your lifestyle and preferences increases the likelihood of consistency. Find a gym in an area you frequent, like your home, work, or church. If you are already in the area, hitting the gym can become an easy habit to add. Also look for a place that feels like you; gyms have different personalities, so find one that matches your personality.

► **INTEGRATE PHYSICAL ACTIVITY INTO DAILY ACTIVITIES:** Find ways to incorporate physical activity into your everyday life. This could include walking or biking to work, taking the stairs instead of the elevator, or doing body-weight exercises while watching TV.

Overcoming Common Challenges in Habit Formation:

► **DEALING WITH LACK OF MOTIVATION:** It's normal to experience days when you're not motivated to work out. On such days, focus on the habit of getting started rather than the intensity of the workout. Often, starting will lead to a more productive workout than anticipated. This is what I called "Turning the Dial" in chapter eight.

- ► **AVOIDING BURNOUT:** To prevent burnout, ensure your fitness routine is not overly taxing or monotonous. Incorporate various exercises, allow for rest days, and adjust the intensity of your workouts as needed.

- ► **HANDLING SETBACKS:** When faced with setbacks, such as missing a workout, practicing self-compassion and avoiding self-criticism is essential. Recognize that setbacks are part of the process and focus on getting back on track with the next planned activity.

Maintaining Long-Term Fitness Habits

Techniques for Sustaining Habits Over Time:

- ► **SET PROGRESSIVE GOALS:** As you become comfortable with your fitness routine, set new, slightly more challenging goals. This keeps the routine engaging and prevents stagnation. The key is to make these goals attainable yet motivating, a concept that is built into many group class gyms, such as CrossFit. Learning new skills or increasing personal records can help build habits.

► **TRACK YOUR PROGRESS:** Keeping a record of your fitness journey, whether through a journal, app, or social media, can be highly motivating. Seeing your progress over time reinforces the habit and encourages you to continue.

► **REGULARLY REVIEW AND ADJUST YOUR ROUTINE:** As your fitness level, interests, and life circumstances change, your fitness routine should evolve, too. Periodically review and adjust your routine. This keeps it relevant and exciting, which is crucial for long-term commitment.

Adapting Habits to Changing Circumstances

Life is dynamic, and your fitness habits should be flexible enough to accommodate changes. Be prepared to modify your routine as needed, whether due to a change in work schedule, an injury, or a new family commitment. Flexibility in your approach to fitness ensures that you can maintain your habits even when circumstances change. Injuries will happen, but I know of no injuries that require ending your fitness journey.

The Role of Community and Support Systems

► **SEEK SUPPORT FROM FRIENDS, FAMILY, OR FITNESS COMMUNITIES:** Sharing your fitness journey with others can provide a sense of accountability and motivation. Whether it's a workout buddy, a fitness class, or an online community, having support can make the journey more enjoyable and sustainable. I shared more on this in chapter seven.

► **LEVERAGE SOCIAL MEDIA FOR MOTIVATION AND ACCOUNTABILITY:** Social media can be a powerful tool for sustaining fitness habits. Following fitness influencers, joining fitness groups, or posting progress can keep you engaged and motivated.

Maintaining long-term fitness requires setting short- and long-term goals, tracking progress, adapting to changes, and seeking support. With these strategies, you can ensure that your fitness habits become a lasting part of your lifestyle.

Habits are more than just repeated actions; they are complex processes involving neurological and psychological elements. Understanding how habits form in the brain and the psychological principles that sustain them can empower us to create lasting fitness routines.

Building and maintaining fitness habits is a journey that goes beyond mere physical transformation. It's about creating a lifestyle that nurtures your physical, mental, and emotional health and allows you to care for those around you. The journey will have its challenges, but the rewards of perseverance, improved health, and well-being are immeasurable.

Remember, the goal is not to be perfect but to be consistent. Celebrate the small victories, learn from the setbacks, and stay committed to your journey toward a healthier, happier you. Keep pushing forward, stay patient, and trust the process. Your fitness journey is unique, and so is your path to forming and maintaining these life-changing habits.

CHAPTER 10

THE ROLE OF REST AND RECOVERY

In a world that often glorifies "the grind" and "getting shit done," the roles of rest and recovery in maintaining health and enhancing longevity are frequently underestimated. Rest is not merely a passive state of inactivity; it is an active physiological process crucial for an individual's physical and mental well-being. Recovery, particularly from physical exertion, is vital to any health regimen, allowing the body to heal, rebuild, and strengthen.

This chapter delves into the importance of rest and recovery, drawing upon insights from David A. Sinclair's influential book *Lifespan: Why We Age - and Why We Don't Have To*, which sheds light on the connection between rest and cellular health. We will explore the science behind rest and recovery and provide practical advice for improving sleep and incorporating effective recovery techniques into your daily routine.

Understanding and applying these principles is vital to achieving a balanced, healthy lifestyle and extending your lifespan. Because as you know, you are no use to anyone if you are not around.

Definition and Significance

Rest and recovery are often used interchangeably, but they hold distinct meanings. Rest generally refers to the cessation of strenuous physical or mental activity, allowing the body and mind to relax. On the other hand, recovery is the process through which the body repairs itself after physical exertion, stress, or injury.

Rest and recovery are very important. They are fundamental for maintaining physical health, enhancing mental clarity, and improving overall well-being. During rest, the body conserves energy, repairs tissue, and strengthens the immune system. At the same time, the mind consolidates memories and processes information.

Different Types of Rest and Their Benefits:

► **PHYSICAL REST:** This involves giving the body a break from physical activities. It helps in muscle repair, reduces fatigue, and prevents overuse injuries. Physical rest can be active, like light walking or yoga, or passive, like sleeping or sitting.

► **MENTAL REST:** Mental rest is crucial for cognitive functions. It involves activities that divert the mind from stressful thoughts, such as meditation, reading, or hobbies. Mental rest helps reduce stress, improve concentration, and boost mood.

► **EMOTIONAL REST:** Emotional rest entails stepping away from emotional stressors and engaging in activities that promote emotional well-being, like spending time with loved ones or practicing mindfulness.

► **SOCIAL REST:** Social rest means taking a break from social interactions, especially if they are draining or stressful. It's essential for recharging and maintaining a healthy social life balance.

Key Concepts Related to Rest and Aging

In *Lifespan*,[5] David A. Sinclair presents ground-breaking insights into the aging process and how various lifestyle factors, including rest, play a crucial role. Sinclair emphasizes that aging is not just an inevitable decline but a process that our daily choices can influence. One of the key concepts he discusses is the role of rest in regulating cellular health and longevity.

How Rest Impacts Cellular Health and Longevity

Sinclair explores the idea that rest periods are essential for cellular repair and rejuvenation. During rest, the body engages in several critical processes, such as clearing cellular waste, repairing DNA damage, and reducing oxidative stress. These processes are vital for maintaining cellular health, impacting overall aging and longevity.

He also discusses the concept of hormesis, the idea that exposing the body to periods of stress followed by rest can enhance its ability to cope with stress and potentially slow the aging process. This is where the balance between activity and rest becomes crucial. Rest allows the body to recover from stressors, strengthening cellular resilience.

Sinclair's research suggests that improving the quality of rest and recovery can have significant anti-aging effects. By ensuring adequate rest, we can help maintain the health of our cells, which is vital in prolonging a healthy lifespan.

The Science of Sleep and Recovery

Next, we will delve deeper into the science of sleep and its role in physical and mental recovery. Understanding the intricate relationship between sleep and the body's repair processes will further illustrate the importance of rest in maintaining long-term health and wellness.

Sleep Helps Both Physical and Mental Health

Sleep is not just a period of rest; it's an active state where numerous vital processes occur. It plays a crucial role in physical health by aiding in the repair and regeneration of tissues, strengthening the immune system, and balancing hormones. Sleep also contributes significantly to brain health, facilitating memory consolidation, cognitive function, and emotional regulation.

When we are in the deeper stages of sleep, our body releases growth hormone. This hormone plays a crucial role in muscle growth and repair, and it is vital for people who exercise regularly, as it helps in the recovery of muscles and strengthens them for future physical activity.

How Sleep Affects the Body's Repair Processes

During sleep, the body undergoes several critical restorative processes for maintaining good health. One of these processes is autophagy, where cells get rid of damaged components, helping to prevent the buildup of cellular debris that can cause aging and disease.

Sleep also plays a significant role in brain health. The brain's glymphatic system becomes more active during sleep, clearing out waste products like beta-amyloid, which is linked to Alzheimer's disease. This detoxification process is essential for maintaining cognitive health and function.

However, inadequate sleep can disrupt these repair processes, leading to several health issues. These issues range from impaired cognitive function and mood disorders to an increased risk of chronic diseases like diabetes and heart disease.

Strategies to Improve Sleep Quality:

- ► **MAINTAIN A CONSISTENT SLEEP SCHEDULE:** Your body needs routine. Going to bed and waking up at the same time every day, even on weekends, helps regulate your body's clock and improves the quality of your sleep.

► **ESTABLISH A BEDTIME RITUAL:** Having a calming routine before bed can signal your body that it's time to rest. This could include reading, showering, or meditation.

► **OPTIMIZE YOUR SLEEP ENVIRONMENT:** The environment in which you sleep can significantly affect the quality of your rest. Make sure your bedroom is cool, quiet, and dark. Investing in a comfortable mattress and pillows can also make a significant difference.

Importance of Sleep Hygiene

Good sleep hygiene involves practices and habits conducive to sleeping well regularly. This includes:

► **LIMITING EXPOSURE TO SCREENS BEFORE BEDTIME:** The blue light emitted by phones, tablets, and computers can interfere with your body's production of melatonin, the hormone that regulates sleep. Try to avoid screens at least an hour before bed.

► **WATCHING YOUR DIET:** Avoid large meals, caffeine, and alcohol close to bedtime, as they can disrupt sleep. Instead, opt for a light snack if you're slightly hungry.

► **GETTING REGULAR PHYSICAL ACTIVITY:** Regular exercise can promote better sleep, helping you to fall asleep faster and enjoy deeper sleep. However, vigorous exercise should be avoided close to bedtime, as it might have the opposite effect.

Improving Sleep Through Mindfulness and Relaxation Techniques:

► **MINDFULNESS MEDITATION:** Mindfulness meditation can help calm your mind and reduce sleep-disturbing anxiety and stress. Various apps and online resources are available to guide you through mindfulness practices suitable for bedtime.

► **DEEP BREATHING OR PROGRESSIVE MUSCLE RELAXATION:** Techniques like deep breathing or progressive muscle relaxation can reduce stress and induce relaxation, making it easier to fall asleep.

Recovery Techniques Beyond Sleep

Active Recovery:

- ► **LIGHT EXERCISE:** On rest days, consider engaging in light exercise like walking, swimming, or yoga. These activities increase blood flow, aiding muscle recovery and reducing soreness without putting excessive strain on the body.

- ► **STRETCHING AND FOAM ROLLING:** Incorporating stretching and foam rolling into your recovery routine can help release muscle tightness and improve flexibility. These practices can also enhance blood circulation, which is vital for transporting nutrients to the muscles for repair and recovery.

Meditation and Mindfulness:

- ► **MENTAL RECOVERY:** Just as physical recovery is essential, so is mental recovery. Meditation and mindfulness can help lower stress levels, improve sleep quality, and improve overall mental well-being. These techniques allow the mind to rest and rejuvenate, which is essential for maintaining motivation and focus in your fitness journey.

▶ **GUIDED RELAXATION:** Techniques such as guided imagery or relaxation exercises can greatly reduce mental fatigue and enhance overall recovery.

Nutrition and Hydration:

▶ **PROPER NUTRITION:** What you eat significantly affects how quickly and effectively your body recovers. Consuming a balanced diet rich in protein, healthy fats, and carbohydrates aids in muscle repair and energy replenishment. Remember to include plenty of fruits and vegetables for their vitamins and minerals.

▶ **STAY HYDRATED:** Adequate hydration is crucial for recovery. Water supports every metabolic function and nutrient transfer in the body and is essential for efficient recovery.

Encouraging a Holistic Approach to Rest and Recovery

Embracing a holistic approach to rest and recovery is essential for a healthy lifestyle. It's not just about how much you exercise or how busy you are; it's about balancing activity with adequate rest and recovery time. This balance is key to maintaining physical health, mental clarity, and emotional well-being.

Remember, taking time to rest and recover is not a sign of weakness; it's a crucial aspect of a sustainable health regimen. By incorporating these practices into your life, you're enhancing your immediate health and investing in your long-term well-being and longevity.

As you integrate these insights and strategies into your life, celebrate the small steps you take towards a more rested, healthier you. Your journey to putting fitness first is not just about the physical milestones but also about learning to listen to your body and giving it the rest and care it deserves.

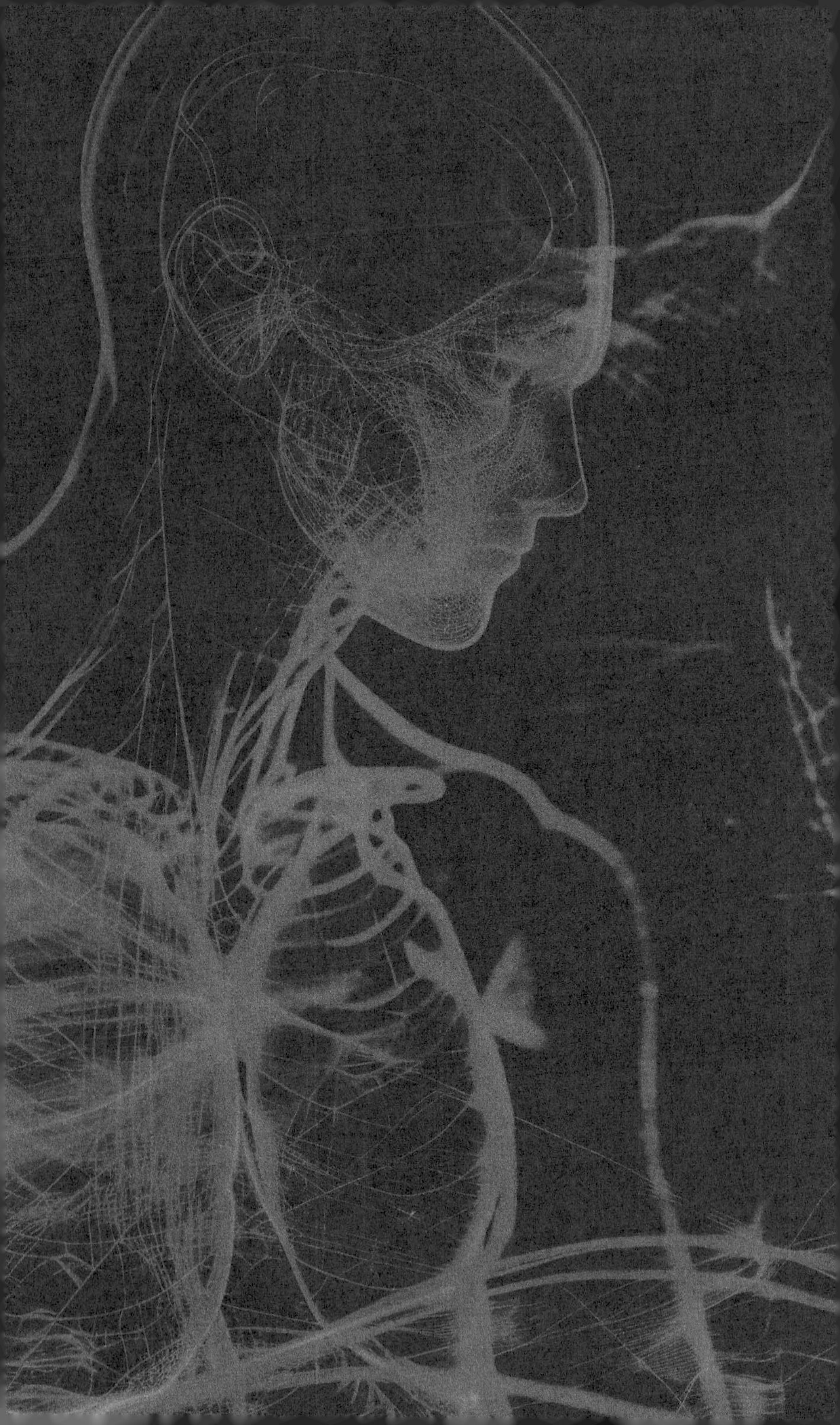

PROGRESS AND BEYOND

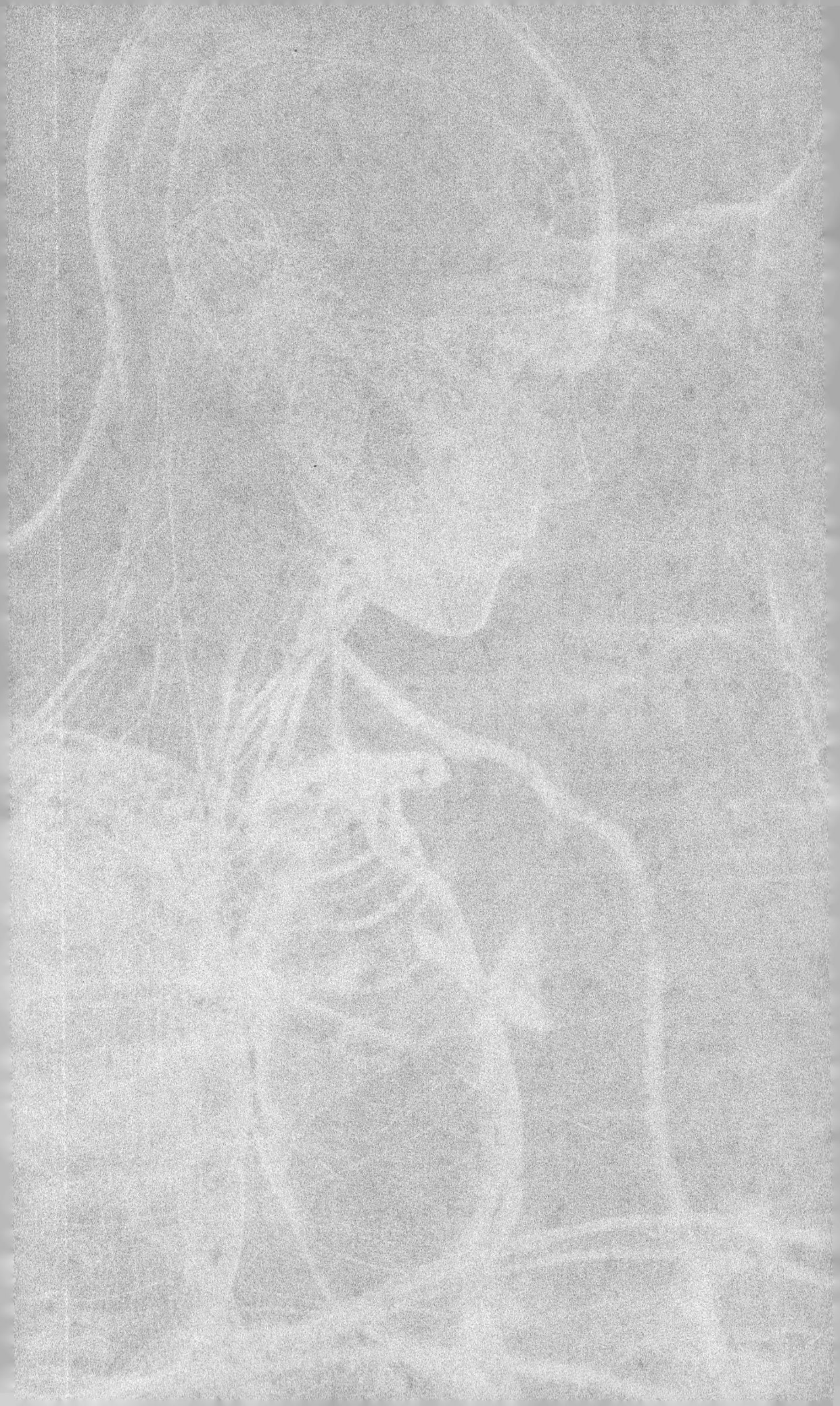

CHAPTER 11

TRACKING YOUR FITNESS JOURNEY

Have you ever started a fitness journey and felt like you were running in circles? You're not alone. Imagine training for months and not knowing if you're any closer to your goals—frustrating, right? Sometimes, the mirror and scale don't tell the whole story. That's where tracking progress comes in, turning guesswork into science.

Tracking your fitness isn't just about flaunting those numbers on social media (though let's be honest, it feels pretty good). It's about understanding your body, recognizing your achievements, and steering your fitness in the right direction.

The Science of Tracking

Why do we even bother tracking our fitness progress? Beyond the obvious ego boost when those numbers are inching in the right direction, science backs the benefits of tracking.

Psychological Benefits of Tracking

First off, tracking progress is like giving yourself a high-five; it boosts motivation and self-esteem. It's a mini celebration each time you log a faster mile or a heavier lift. Psychology tells us that these small victories release dopamine, our feel-good neurotransmitter. It's like your brain saying, "Heck yeah, let's do that again!"

Research has proven that people who track their progress are more likely to improve. A study by Dominican University of California[6] found that those who write down their goals and share weekly updates are 33% more successful than those who don't. That's a significant advantage just from jotting down a few notes.

Hitting Targets and Raising Bars

Goal tracking isn't only about hitting targets; it's also about knowing when to raise the bar. Without tracking, you're just shooting in the dark. With tracking, you know exactly when it's time to push a bit harder.

Remember, fitness isn't a one-size-fits-all journey. What works for your gym buddy might not work for you. Tracking helps you figure out your unique path. It's sort of like detective work, but instead of solving crimes, you're unlocking your fitness potential.

Picture this: Jenny, a friend of mine, started her fitness journey with all the enthusiasm in the world. But, three months in, she's about to throw in the towel, feeling like she's gotten nowhere. Sound familiar? But here's the key: Jenny wasn't tracking her progress. When she finally started logging her workouts and diet, she was shocked to learn that she was improving steadily, just not in the way she had expected.

Or take Mark, who thought he was doing everything right but just wasn't seeing results. Once he started tracking, he realized he was overestimating his activity level and underestimating his calorie intake-a classic mistake! He made adjustments and started seeing progress.

These stories highlight the "aha" moments that come from tracking. Just like with putting together a puzzle, the picture gets more evident with each piece. You're able to start connecting the dots between your actions and the results you see—or don't see.

Think about it: How often have you wondered if you're on the right track? Tracking gives you that assurance—or a gentle nudge to change course.

Tools and Techniques for Tracking Fitness

Tracking your fitness journey doesn't mean just scribbling numbers in a notebook anymore (though if that's your jam, more power to you). We're living in the age of technology where tracking options are just a tap away.

Wearable Tech and Apps

There are several options in the form of wearable tech, such as fitness trackers, smartwatches, and heart rate monitors. These gadgets are akin to having a mini personal trainer on your wrist. They track everything from your steps and heart rate to your sleep patterns. And let's not overlook the multitude of fitness apps available. Whether you're into running, weightlifting, yoga, or general fitness, there's an app that's perfect for you.

Visualizing Your Progress

Most fitness apps will give you clear visuals of your progress. There's something incredibly satisfying about seeing your efforts translated into colorful graphs that trend upwards.

Imagine a line graph showing your running pace over the months, each dip and rise telling its own story, or a bar chart displaying your increasing strength training weights. It's like watching your superhero transformation in real-time.

Old-School Methods

If tech isn't your thing, there's always the old-school method. A simple journal can be just as effective. Write down your workouts, how you felt, and what you ate—it's all valuable data. Plus, putting pen to paper can be quite therapeutic.

Integrating Tracking into Your Routine

The key is to make tracking a seamless part of your routine. It shouldn't feel like a chore. Find a method that works for you, something that you can stick with. Remember, consistency is king.

Interpreting Data and Adjusting Goals

So, you've been diligently tracking your progress—kudos to you! But now you're staring at this data, wondering, "What on earth does this all mean?" Let's break it down.

Making Sense of the Numbers

As I mentioned earlier, tracking and interpreting your fitness data is like being a detective. You're looking for clues and patterns. Did your running times improve after you switched up your training routine? Did you lift heavier after adding more protein to your diet? These insights are gold; they help you understand what's working and what's not.

Listening to What the Data Tells You

It's crucial to listen to what the data is telling you. If you're consistently missing your targets, this might be a sign to reevaluate your goals. Maybe they were too ambitious. Maybe your nutrition is off. Maybe your recovery is not right. Maybe you need to make adjustments to your lifestyle as well as your exercise habits. It's okay to adjust your goals. It's not admitting defeat; it's being smart and realistic.

When to Push and When to Pivot

Your data can also tell you when to push harder or switch things up. If you've been comfortably hitting your targets for a while, it's time to challenge yourself more. On the flip side, if you're constantly feeling burnt out, it might be time to dial it back a notch.

Remember, tracking isn't about obsessing over numbers; it's about understanding your journey, celebrating your successes, and learning from the not-so-great days.

It's Your Story—Track It Your Way

Think of tracking as writing your fitness story. Each entry, each data point, is a sentence in your ongoing narrative. And the best part? You're both the author and the protagonist. Whether you prefer high-tech gadgets or the old pen-and-paper method, find your style and stick with it.

Embrace the Journey

Let's be honest: The path to fitness isn't always smooth. There will be days when you feel like a champ and days when you'd rather be anywhere but the gym. That's normal. What matters is that you keep showing up. And with your trusty tracking tools, you'll have a clear picture of how far you've come.

You Are Not the Numbers

Don't let the numbers define you. They're just signposts along the way, helping you navigate your fitness journey. The true measure of success is how you feel: stronger, healthier, and more alive.

Track your progress, make adjustments, and most importantly, enjoy the ride. You're doing something meaningful for yourself and those you love, and that is worth celebrating every step of the way.

CHAPTER 12

TIME MANAGEMENT AND GOAL SETTING

Have you ever felt like there are just not enough hours in the day, especially for squeezing in a workout? You're not alone. Managing time can often feel like walking two dogs while attending a Zoom meeting for work. Time management is tricky but not impossible—and when it comes to fitness, it's a game-changer.

Why bother with scheduling workouts or setting fitness goals, you ask? Without a plan, your fitness journey is like a ship without a rudder—aimlessly drifting. Let's face it: "I'll work out tomorrow" often turns into "I'll never work out." And that is just not acceptable. You have important things to do, and the people you love need you to be at your best.

The Importance of Scheduling Workouts

Imagine it's Monday. You're pumped and ready to hit the gym "sometime later today." Fast forward to ten p.m.—you're sprawled on the couch, binge-watching your favorite series, and the thought of going to the gym is a distant memory. Sound familiar? That's exactly why scheduling your workouts is a must.

Why Scheduling Is Key

Scheduling workouts is about making a commitment, a nonnegotiable appointment with your health. It's like setting a meeting with your boss: You wouldn't dream of skipping that, would you? When workouts are a fixed part of your calendar, they're harder to brush off. When they are thought of as nonnegotiable, they get done.

A Tale Of Two Gym-Goers

Let's talk about Jim and Pam. They work in an office—you know which one I am talking about. Jim's approach is all about "fitting in a workout when I feel like it." Pam, on the other hand, has her workouts scheduled like clockwork. Guess who's more consistent and seeing better results? You got it: Pam. While Jim's good intentions often get lost in the chaos of daily life, Pam's structured approach keeps her on track.

Making It Work For You

You might be thinking, "But my schedule is as predictable as a plot twist in Yellowstone." Fear not. The trick is to be realistic. Can't do an hour? Go for a brisk twenty-minute walk. Don't have time in the mornings? Schedule your workouts for the evening. Find slots in your day that work for you and stick to them.

Setting Realistic Fitness Goals

Ever set a fitness goal so high you forgot what you were thinking about when you set it? We've all been there, aiming for the fitness equivalent of climbing Everest when we've barely conquered the local hill. This is where the art of setting realistic goals comes into play.

The Goldilocks Of Goals

Your fitness goals should be like Goldilocks's porridge—just right. Not too easy or hard, but challenging enough to push you without setting you up for disappointment. Setting attainable goals keeps you motivated. There's nothing like the thrill of smashing a goal to spur you on to the next one. If you need a reminder on how to set realistic goals, head back to chapter eight.

I'll tell you about a friend who decided to "get in shape" for a wedding. With no clear goal, her efforts were scattered, to say the least. Fast-forward to when she set a specific target: to be fit (deadlift 185 pounds) and confident (fit into her favorite dress) by the wedding date. Suddenly, her workouts had a purpose, and her diet had direction. She ended up illuminating the wedding with positive energy and was strong enough to help carry Uncle Brad to his room after he had a bit too much fun.

Time Management Strategies

Once you've got your goals lined up, finding time for them may remain a significant struggle. Time management is the secret sauce for squeezing in those workouts and making them count. Let's explore some strategies for making time your ally:

- ▶ **PLAN LIKE A PRO:** Ever heard Benjamin Franklin's saying, "If you fail to plan, you plan to fail"? It's cliché but true. Take a few minutes each week to plan your workouts. Treat them like important appointments—because they are. Whether it's a thirty-minute home workout or a gym session, ink it into your calendar. Your workouts should be scheduled just like everything else necessary in your life. If they are currently not on your calendar, put them in. This is step one. Fitness first means that you put your workouts in first.

► **PRIORITIZE YOUR PRIORITIES:** Here's a no-brainer: Prioritize your fitness goals. It's easy to let exercise slip to the bottom of your to-do list, but remember, health is wealth. Sometimes, this might mean saying no to a Netflix marathon or waking up earlier. Tough love, but your future self and those depending on you will thank you.

► **THE ART OF MULTITASKING:** Who says you can't mix business with pleasure? If you're strapped for time, get creative. How about a walking meeting? Or catching up with friends on a hike? The idea is to make fitness a part of your lifestyle, not an afterthought.

► **SHORT AND SWEET:** No time for a full workout? No problem. Focus on the quality of your workout, not just the duration. Research shows that even short bursts of exercise, like high-intensity interval training (HIIT), can be highly effective. A focused twenty-minute session beats an hour of going through the motions.

► **EMBRACE FLEXIBILITY:** As Bruce Lee said, "Be like water." If an unexpected commitment pops up, don't sweat it. Shuffle your workout schedule around. The key is to adapt, not abandon.

Here's a scenario: Alex thinks he has no time for exercise. Then he starts cycling to work. Boom—cardio ticked off the list. Next, he begins using his lunch breaks for quick gym sessions. Suddenly, he is the guy who "has time for everything."

Balancing Fitness With Everyday Life

Juggling fitness and life's endless curveballs—sounds like a circus act, right? But it's doable with a bit of finesse and balance. Let's talk about how to weave fitness into the fabric of your everyday life without it feeling like a chore:

► **INTEGRATION OVER ISOLATION:** Think of fitness as an integral part of your day, not something you do in isolation. Got kids?

Turn playtime into a mini workout session; they will love it, probably more than you do. Waiting for the pasta to boil? Time for some kitchen counter push-ups. Look for opportunities in your daily routine and capitalize on them.

▶ **THE EARLY BIRD OR THE NIGHT OWL:** Identify when you're at your peak. Are you the early bird who catches the worm with a sunrise jog? Or the night owl who hits the gym when others hit the sack? Tailoring your workout schedule to your natural rhythm can make a difference.

▶ **THE POWER OF ROUTINE:** Consistency is king. Carve out a routine and stick to it. The more you ingrain fitness into your daily life, the less you'll have to battle with willpower. It's like brushing your teeth—you just do it.

Let's look at an example: Sara has a full-time job, two kids, and a dog that needs walking. She swapped out her coffee breaks for quick stair climbs and turned dog-walking into a power-walking session. Time management is all about finding those pockets of time and making them count.

We've navigated time management and goal setting in the fitness world. Remember, it's not about having time but making time. With a bit of planning, prioritizing, and a dash of creativity, fitting fitness into your busy schedule is not just a dream, but a doable reality.

Remember Jim and Pam's approaches to fitness and Alex's cycling-to-work revelation? Let these stories be your inspiration. Whether carving out time for a quick workout or setting SMART goals, every step counts. You're not just working out; you're building a lifestyle that harmonizes your health with your hectic schedule. The people around you are counting on you.

Make It Work

Go ahead and schedule those workouts, set those goals, and find that sweet spot in your day. It's all about balance, consistency, and a little fun. Here's to managing your time like a pro and putting fitness first.

CHAPTER 13

OVERCOMING CHALLENGES

Ever felt like life just threw you a curveball when you were expecting a fastball? Welcome to humanity. Overcoming challenges is part of everyone's story. Still, sometimes, it feels like you're in an obstacle course race you didn't sign up for. But you are not living an abnormally difficult life—this is just life.

This chapter delves deep into setbacks and how to overcome them like a "Fitness First" pro, whether you're struggling to stick to your fitness routine, facing roadblocks in personal projects, or dealing with day-to-day hiccups.

Life's a game of whack-a-mole: Just when you think you've got everything under control, a new challenge pops up. But hey, that's what makes life interesting, right? Let's talk about some common setbacks you might face:

- ► **LACK OF MOTIVATION:** It's Monday. You planned to start your new fitness regime, learn a new skill, or get up early. But somehow, you can't muster the energy. Sound familiar? Motivation is a flakey friend.

- ► **TIME MANAGEMENT WOES:** There's so much to do, yet so little time. Managing a full-time job, family responsibilities, and personal goals can feel like juggling with too many balls in the air.

- ► **FEAR OF FAILURE:** This sneaky little gremlin sits on your shoulder, whispering, "What if you fail?" It's often one of the biggest hurdles in starting or continuing a journey towards a goal.

- ► **INJURIES:** Things happen. The key to success with injuries is to continue to do something. I have yet to see an injury that requires someone to stop all activities. If your doctor tells you to stop going to the gym, get a new doctor.

Imagine that Jane starts her fitness journey with gusto but soon hits a wall. Her motivation wanes, her schedule gets chaotic, and the fear of not seeing results creeps in. Her story is not unique—it's as old as time.

Turning the Page

But here's the thing: Setbacks are just plot twists in your story. They're not the end. Recognizing and planning for these common obstacles is the first step in overcoming them. Next, we'll dive into how shifting your mindset and attitude can be a turning point in this battle.

Mindset and Attitude Adjustment

The mind is a powerful thing. Its power can work for you and against you. It's like a supercomputer that sometimes needs a bit of reprogramming. When overcoming challenges, half the battle is won in your head. Let's look at ways to "reboot and update" our mindset.

The Positivity Switch

First, flip the positivity switch. It's easy to drown in a glass-half-empty mindset, but what if we start looking at setbacks as opportunities? Missed a workout? That's a chance to double down tomorrow. Is your life going differently than planned? Time to reset. It's okay. We'll go again tomorrow.

Embrace the "Yet"

"Yet" is a mighty word and highly underrated. It's full of possibilities. Can't do a pull-up? You can't do it yet. Haven't finished that big project? You haven't finished it yet. "Yet" implies that you're on your way, and that's a powerful mindset shift.

The Learning Lens

View every setback through a learning lens. Ask yourself, "What can I learn from this?" This approach turns obstacles into lessons, not road-blocks. Get to this mindset as quickly as possible.

Building Resilience Through Habits and Routine

Building resilience is like constructing a fortress; it doesn't happen overnight. It's forged through consistent habits and routines that keep you grounded, no matter how strong the storm. So, how do we build it?

▶ **DAILY HABITS FOR THE WIN:** It's the little things that add up. Start with small, daily habits that contribute to your goals. This could be as simple as waking up thirty minutes earlier for a quick workout or dedicating fifteen minutes daily to learning a new skill. Over time, these habits become the building blocks of resilience.

- ► **ROUTINE IS YOUR ALLY:** Establish a routine that aligns with your goals and stick to it. Routines provide structure, reduce the mental load of decision-making, and make challenging tasks more manageable. When your actions are aligned with your routine, tackling obstacles becomes part of your daily flow, rather than an insurmountable challenge.

- ► **FLEXIBILITY WITHIN STRUCTURE:** While routines are great, too much rigidity can be a downfall. Be flexible and willing to adjust your routine as needed. Life is unpredictable; pivoting while maintaining the core of your routine is critical to resilience.

Here's a scenario: Sarah has a strict workout routine. When an injury sidelines her, she doesn't give up. Instead, she adjusts her routine to include low-impact exercises and focuses more on nutrition. Her resilience isn't in sticking to the routine but in her ability to adapt it to her new situation.

Remember, setbacks are not roadblocks; they're stepping stones to success. By breaking down your goals, embracing routines, and staying flexible, you're equipping yourself with the tools to overcome just about anything life throws your way.

Also keep in mind the power of a good coach. They're like the Gandalf to your Frodo, guiding you through the perils of Middle-earth—or you know, your fitness journey. A coach can provide the wisdom, encouragement, and accountability you need to conquer your personal Mount Doom.

Next time you face a challenge, take a deep breath, remember these tips, and tackle it head-on. You've got this! Every challenge you overcome gains you more knowledge and earned confidence, which you can share with those around you.

GETTING STARTED— FIRST STEPS TO REAL CHANGE

Now what?

Now that you've read the book and geared up your mindset, what are the next steps?

1. **FIGURE OUT YOUR REASON—YOUR WHY:** Complete the "Fitness First: Real Why Worksheet." Who will be affected by you meeting your goal? What else will change? If your goal is a number, time, or weight on the scale, go back and reread chapter four.

2. **BREAK IT DOWN:** Big goals can be overwhelming. The trick? Break them into smaller, more manageable chunks. I also talked about this in chapter four. Want to run a marathon?

Start by running a mile, then five, and so on. It's like eating an elephant one bite at a time—not that you'd want to eat an elephant, but you get the analogy.

3. **SCHEDULE, SCHEDULE, SCHEDULE:** Remember, what gets scheduled gets done. Carve out specific times for your tasks or workouts. Treat these slots like important appointments. Do not cancel unless absolutely necessary.

4. **ACCOUNTABILITY PARTNERS:** Having someone to share your journey with can be a huge boost. This could be a workout buddy, a colleague, or a family member. When someone else is counting on you, skipping out becomes much harder.

5. **EMBRACE TECHNOLOGY:** Nowadays, there's an app for almost everything. Find one and use it to your advantage. Fitness trackers, reminder apps, or goal-setting tools can be incredibly helpful for keeping you on track.

6. **HIRE A COACH:** Sometimes, you need that extra push of an expert to guide you, hold you accountable, and provide tailored advice. That's where hiring a coach comes

in. A coach can offer a fresh perspective, specialized knowledge, and the motivation you need to overcome your hurdles. Plus, it's an investment in yourself—and what's more important than that? If you need to get somewhere fast, you hire a guide.

Imagine you're learning to play the guitar. You hit a wall and can't seem to get past it. Now, picture having a music coach who provides you with personalized tips, encouragement, and accountability. Consider how much of a difference this would make. Coaching is the fastest way to achieve something new, and fitness is no different. Hiring a coach is also incredibly helpful if you aim to become fitter for all the right reasons but have not done "fitness" before. Find a good coach to lead you to your best and most impactful self.

LIFELONG FITNESS GUIDE

Fitness is a lifelong journey, evolving with us from playful childhood runs to mindful movements in our golden years. Let's explore how we can embrace a "Fitness First" lifestyle at any age, making each step and stretch a celebration of life's vibrant journey.

Kids: Planting the Seeds of Movement

Before the teenage years come knocking, there's a magical window where movement is a natural part of a child's world. This isn't about grooming future athletes; it's about instilling a love for being active. Whether it's soccer for kindergarteners, an impromptu dance party in the living room, or a family nature hike, the goal is simple: Movement should be synonymous with fun.

Coaching the Little Champions

As parents, guardians, or coaches, our role isn't just to instruct and inspire. The focus should be on creating a joyful atmosphere where movement is a game and teamwork is celebrated. This early foundation sets the stage for a positive relationship with fitness, built on smiles and sweat in equal measure.

A World of Movement: Beyond Sports

Not every child dreams of scoring goals or running races, and that's perfectly okay. Fitness isn't one-size-fits-all; it's a spectrum of activities. Encourage walks to talk about their day, bike rides to explore, or even help with gardening. The key is to make movement a natural part of their day, as regular as their favorite bedtime story.

18-25 Years Old, Navigating Life's Transitions Through Fitness

The Prime of Youth: Balancing Fun and Fitness

In the whirlwind of young adulthood, sports and physical activities often remain central, but it's crucial to maintain a balance. This age isn't just about scoring goals or crossing finish lines; it's about understanding that fitness is a companion that helps navigate life's changes. Whether in college, starting a new job, or exploring relationships, keeping fit can be your anchor.

Beyond the Field:
Exploring Diverse Fitness Avenues

Not everyone is a sports enthusiast, and that's the beauty of this age: exploration. Group fitness classes offer choices from high-energy boot camps to serene yoga sessions. The aim is to move, discover new passions, and understand your body's needs. These classes aren't just workouts; they're learning hubs where fitness becomes a lifestyle, not just an activity.

The Long Game: Building Lifelong Fitness Habits

This period is crucial for establishing habits that echo into your future. It's not about hitting the gym with an all-or-nothing attitude; it's about consistency and making intelligent choices. Fitness during these years is like planting a garden: It requires patience, care, and a bit of trial and error. The goal is to wake up at twenty-five not lamenting lost time, but celebrating a foundation of health that is ready to support life's next adventures.

25-35 Years Old: Solidifying Habits Amidst Life's Hustle

Settling In: The Decade of Decision-Making

Life in your late twenties and early thirties is often synonymous with settling into a lifestyle. Still, it's also a critical time for fitness choices. This decade can set the tone for the next several years, making it imperative to weave fitness into your evolving life narrative. Whether you're experiencing career growth, starting a family, or personal exploration, integrating fitness is less about creating time and more about making it a nonnegotiable part of your schedule.

Finding Your Fitness Groove

This period is perfect for experimenting and finding what resonates with you. It's about exploring different sports, fitness programs, and lifestyle choices that align with your evolving priorities and responsibilities. Remember, fitness is a personal journey that should reflect your interests, goals, and life circumstances.

Prioritizing Health: The Real Wealth

Amidst the bustle of career and family life, it's easy to put fitness on the back burner; however, this is the time to reinforce that your health is your most vital asset. Engaging with a fitness coach or joining a community-based gym can be instrumental in keeping you on track. A trainer will help you navigate your fitness journey amidst the complexities of adult life.

35-45 Years Old: Balancing Fitness With Family and Career

Embracing Change: Fitness as a Family Affair

This phase of life often finds many juggling family responsibilities and career aspirations. Fitness during these years can become a shared activity, not just an individual pursuit. Movement is often integrated into family life, whether weekend cycling trips, playing sports together, or simply opting for active vacations. Fitness becomes a bonding experience, enriching not just your health but also your family dynamics.

The Career-Fitness Balance

Professionally, you might be reaching your stride, but it's crucial to maintain physical momentum. Exercise during this period isn't just about staying fit; it's about managing stress, enhancing mental clarity, and maintaining the energy needed to excel in your career. This is also the time to recognize the importance of muscle maintenance and incorporate strength training into your routine.

Adapting to Your Body's Needs

As your body changes, so should your fitness routine. Rather than cling to past fitness glories, adapt to your body's needs. This might mean switching high-impact workouts for lower-impact alternatives like swimming, cycling, or pilates. The focus should be on sustaining mobility, strength, and endurance, ensuring you're as agile in your daily life as you are in your fitness pursuits.

45-55 Years Old: Nurturing Fitness as a Cornerstone of Life

The Critical Decade: Making Fitness Nonnegotiable

In your mid-forties to mid-fifties, fitness transcends being a mere routine; it becomes a cornerstone of your lifestyle. This is when your fitness habits visibly impact your quality of life. It's important to recognize that staying active is not just a choice but a necessity for maintaining health, vitality, and independence.

Embracing Strength and Mobility

Now, more than ever, strength training and maintaining mobility should be critical components of your fitness regimen. If you haven't yet incorporated these into your routine, there is still time to start. Your focus should be on exercises that build muscle, enhance flexibility, and support joint health, ensuring you're as active and agile as possible.

Adjusting Intensity: Smart Fitness Choices

Gone are the days of reckless workouts. Now is the time to pursue fitness with wisdom, focusing on activities that yield maximum benefits with minimal risk. This might mean modifying high-intensity workouts or opting for low-impact alternatives that are kinder to your joints but still challenging enough to keep you fit and energized.

The Role of a Coach: Guided Fitness

Consider working with a fitness coach who understands the nuances of training in this age group. A good coach can help tailor your workouts to suit your body's evolving needs, ensuring you stay on track without risking injury. They can be invaluable in helping you navigate the physical changes that come with this stage of life.

55-75 Years Old and Beyond: Adapting and Thriving in Later Life

The Golden Years: Fitness for Longevity and Joy

As you enter your mid-fifties to seventies and beyond, the focus of fitness shifts toward maintaining independence, enhancing quality of life, and savoring the joy of movement. This isn't about training for marathons or setting personal bests; it's about nurturing a routine that keeps you vibrant, mobile, and engaged in life's daily pleasures.

Exploring New Avenues of Fitness

This is an ideal time to explore gentler, yet effective forms of exercise. Activities like yoga, swimming, light martial arts, and even walking golf courses (ditch the cart!) offer fitness benefits while being kind to your body. The goal is to find activities you enjoy that keep you motivated and consistent in your fitness journey.

Strength Training: A Nonnegotiable

Contrary to popular belief, strength training remains crucial during these years. It's not about lifting heavy weights but maintaining muscle mass, bone density, and overall body strength. Tailored programs focusing on moderate weight training can help counteract age-related muscle loss and keep your metabolism active.

The Power of a Supportive Community

Joining fitness groups or classes tailored to your age can provide appropriate exercise routines and a sense of community and camaraderie. Being part of a group can be a powerful motivator, making fitness a social and enjoyable part of your routine.

Embracing a Holistic Approach

This period calls for a holistic approach to health, where fitness is just one part of the bigger picture. Attention to nutrition, mental health, and regular health check-ups become equally important. Remember, it's not only about adding years to your life, but adding life to your years.

A Lifelong Fitness Journey

One truth is clear: Fitness is not a phase but a lifelong companion. From the playful activities of childhood to the mindful movements of our later years, fitness adapts and grows with us. Each decade brings challenges and opportunities, but the underlying message remains the same—movement is essential.

Regardless of age, the language of movement is universal. It speaks of strength, resilience, and the joy of living. Whether you're a young adult discovering the thrill of a new sport, a busy parent juggling family and career, or enjoying the wisdom of your later years, fitness can enhance your life.

FITNESS FIRST: MORE THAN A MOTTO

Choosing a "Fitness First" mindset means prioritizing health and well-being over all else, regardless of any challenges that come your way. It's about being intentional in your decisions and ensuring they align with maintaining an active lifestyle. Remember that it's never too late to begin, and the rewards extend beyond physical health.

A Legacy of Health, Happiness, and Leadership

Putting fitness first is more than just engaging in physical activities; it's about leading a healthy and fulfilling life. It's a promise to yourself to live each day with energy and enthusiasm and inspire others to do the same. It's time to view fitness as part of our identity, rather than just something we should do. By doing so, we can enjoy a life full of health and vitality—creating a ripple effect that touches our family, friends, and community.

Remember, you matter to the people around you, and taking care of yourself is essential to be there for them as long as possible. So, lace up your shoes, step onto your mat, dive into the pool, or go for a walk. The magic is in the movement, and the journey is yours to enjoy.

Joshua J. Grenell can be found:
f www.facebook.com/grenell
@joshua_grenell
Website: **JOSHUAGRENELL.COM**

Fitness First
Real Why Worksheet

Answer these questions, and be honest with your responses. Take your time and be curious about yourself. Lastly, be nice to yourself. Your real why may surprise you. There are no wrong answers.

A) Why do you want to improve your health?

B) Why do you want to achieve A?

C) And why is B important?

D) Why will C make a difference?

E) Why will D matter?

F) Who will be affected besides you if you meet this goal?

G) Who else will be positively affected?

References

1. Sung, Yu-Chi, Yi-Hung Liao, Yu-Liang Chen, and Chun-Chung Chou. "Acute Changes in Blood Lipid Profiles and Metabolic Risk Factors in Collegiate Elite Taekwondo Athletes after Short-Term Detraining: A Prospective Insight for Athletic Health Management." Lipids in Health and Disease, 2017. https://lipidworld.biomedcentral.com/counter/pdf/10.1186/s12944-017-0534-2.pdf?site=lipidworld.biomedcentral.com.

2. "'What Is Fitness?' Part 4: The Sickness-Wellness-Fitness Continuum." CrossFit. https://www.crossfit.com/essentials/what-is-fitness-part-4-sickness-wellness-fitness-continuum.

3. "Benefits of Physical Activity." Centers for Disease Control and Prevention, April 24, 2024. https://www.cdc.gov/physical-activity-basics/benefits/?CDC_AAref_Val=https%3A%2F%2Fwww.cdc.gov%2Fphysicalactivity%2Fbasics%2Fpa-health%2Findex.htm.

4. "WHO Guidelines on Physical Activity and Sedentary Behaviour." World Health Organization, 2020. https://iris.who.int/bitstream/handle/10665/337001/9789240014886-eng.pdf.

5. Sinclair, David A. *Lifespan: Why We Age – and Why We Don't Have To*. Atria Books, 2019.

6. Matthews, Gail. "The Impact of Commitment, Accountability, and Written Goals on Goal Achievement." Dominican University of California, 2007. https://scholar.dominican.edu/cgi/viewcontent.cgi?article=1002&context=psychology-faculty-conference-presentations.